ACKNOWLEDGMENTS

My warmest thanks to all the men who shared with me their hearts and souls, their bodies and beds, and their fantasies and desires. Without them, this book wouldn't exist.

I am eternally grateful to Paula Litzky, whose brilliance, savvy, and enthusiasm turned my book fantasies into reality; to Shaye Areheart, for believing in the book so strongly and then making it even better; to the irrepressible Joanna; to Henry D., for his loving support and his poppity-pop-pop ideas; and to Deborah C. for being a great friend, valued advisor, and inspiring Wild Woman.

CONTENTS

"Only the united beat of

sex and heart together can

create ecstasy."

—Anaïs Nin

HOW TO USE THIS BOOK

1. You can read this book straight through from cover to cover, or dip in here and there for a tasty sexual hint whenever the mood strikes you. But whatever you do, be sure to read the first chapter completely. Without these five "Secrets of Great Sex," all the other tips will be much less powerful.

2. It's probably best *not* to show this book to your man. You'll want all these sexy surprises to unfold in your own time, naturally and spontaneously—not because he *expects* them of you.

3. Abandon yourself to your own inventive nature. Use these techniques and ideas as a starting point and then feel free to concoct your own special love treats.

4. Let go of any questions or concerns you may have about why we're figuring out ways to make men happy, instead of the other way around. As a sensitive, caring lover, you already know that truly great sex is more about giving than receiving—especially when you stop to consider that not only are you enjoying these delectable treats yourself, but you're also inspiring your man to do delicious things to you. Sometimes men just don't realize what great lovers they can be until a sexy, loving woman shows them.

5. Know that loving your man—and yourself—is enough. You don't have to perform new and exotic sex tricks every night to be a luscious love goddess. You already are one!

"The potion drunk by lovers

is prepared by no one but themselves.

The potion is the sum

of one's whole existence."

—*Anaïs Nin*

A WORD ABOUT SAFER SEX

It's unfortunate but true that the days of completely carefree sex have come to an end. Though we can be cured of certain sexually transmitted diseases by treatment with penicillin and other antibiotics, these drugs provide no cure for genital herpes or AIDS. So in today's world, part of being a great lover means taking responsibility for protecting yourself and your partner from these very serious diseases.

While total abstinence is one way to protect yourself, it is certainly not an enjoyable solution and is not even necessary. If you and your man have had sex only with each other for at least the past ten years, and neither of you uses drugs intravenously or has had a contaminated blood transfusion, you can safely and happily enjoy any and all of the 203 ways to drive him wild in bed. This will be the case for the vast majority of married couples.

If you and your lover are relatively new to each other, there are still plenty of ways to share some very hot safer sex. Take the time to get to know each other first and establish that you are both concerned about your own and your partner's health and well-being. Don't be shy about saying something like, "With all the talk about herpes and AIDS these days, I really feel concerned about having sex with someone I haven't known well for a very long time, and I'm sure you do, too. I want both of us to feel completely at ease, so why don't we talk a little bit about this." Then you should share with each other your concerns, your current state of health, the extent of your sexual and intravenous drug activity, and what you'd like to do to protect each other. At the very least, *always use a condom*. Make them a part of your lovemaking ritual each and every time. Or perhaps you'll want to wait until you've both been tested for the HIV antibody. (For the test to be effective, you must wait to take it for a period up to six months from your last possible exposure to the HIV virus.)

This may seem awfully clinical and potentially embarrassing, but you're much better off safe than sorry. Neither herpes nor AIDS is curable, and AIDS is a fatal disease. It's easy enough to recognize whether your partner has active herpes lesions; they start out as a small reddened area and then develop into clusters of small white blisters. But it is impossible to determine if your partner carries the HIV virus without proper tests. He may not know it himself. But if he has been sexually active or uses intravenous drugs, the risk is much greater.

There are many excellent books in print that will give

you the basic facts about sexually transmitted diseases and how to protect yourself, and I recommend that you buy at least one and educate yourself. In addition, there is an appendix at the back of this book that offers some basic guidelines for safer sex. *Read it.* Armed with the facts, you'll be able to make informed, intelligent decisions about your sexual activities and determine what precautions you should take. Make this one of the ways you and your lover get to know and care about each other. Be smart. Be firm. Be sure. Then go ahead and enjoy yourself. Having sex with a man you feel comfortable and safe with is the greatest aphrodisiac of all.

"The first and foremost

erogenous zone is

in the mind."

—Richard Alan Miller,

The Magical & Ritual

Use of Aphrodisiacs

1

the

secrets

of

great

sex

$\mathfrak{m}$any years ago, I had a friend named Joanna, who was a great enigma to me. She was extremely plain and had a rather awkward, unappealing body: angular, out of proportion, with small, unattractively shaped breasts and large hips. Although pleasant enough, her personality was nothing out of the ordinary. Her conversation wasn't particularly sparkling and her movements weren't wildly sexual. Yet men—really wonderful men— always swarmed around her. And the lucky few who got her into bed were even more enamored after the heady experience of making love with her. Despite all appearances to the contrary, Joanna was apparently a very sexy woman. What was her secret?

I asked several men who knew her. "I don't know. There's just something about her that's very sexy." "She gives you the impression that she'd be a tigress in bed." "Joanna makes me feel very much like a man, very desirable." "She gives off sexy vibes." "I've never felt so lusted after, so cared for."

I asked Joanna herself. "You know, it never used to be this way," she told me. "I was always the plain Jane and never had many dates. On the rare occasion when I actually went to bed with a man, I didn't know what to do. Then I met a man who treated me like a sex goddess. He acted as if I were the most desirable woman in the world, as if one look from me could drive him wild with desire. In bed, he taught me a lot about both our bodies — how they move, what they feel, how beautiful they are — and I grew to love my body for how it could make me feel instead of being embarrassed about its shortcomings. I learned to see the incredible beauty and sensuous strength in a man's body, too. I began looking at myself in a different way; and men looked at me differently, too. I think they could feel my sexy thoughts and wanted to be part of them. My wonderful man and I parted about a year later, but the erotic feelings he brought to life remained alive. I'm sure that's why men find me desirable — because I *think* I am, I *feel* I am."

This seemed logical, but far too simple. In order to be sexy, all you had to do was *feel* sexy? To become a great lover, you only had to believe that you already were one? What about technique? What about having a luscious body? What about knowing all the most exciting sex tricks? What about vast experience with sexually knowledgeable men? Was "sex appeal" really all in your head?

I decided to try it out for myself. While out walking one day, I silently indulged in one of my favorite fantasies. I imagined that the gorgeous man who lived around the corner was making wild, abandoned love to me. I could "feel" his hot breath and fervent caresses as he whispered impassioned endearments in my ear, telling me how beautiful and sexy I was and how much I turned him on. I imagined that, to him, I was the sexiest woman in the world.

Only half-aware of the real men I was passing in the street, I finally noticed that many of them smiled at me, winked, or at least looked at me with interest. I seemed to be wearing a secret, provocative smile these men found enticing.

I became slightly more sophisticated in my experimentation. Before going out for my man-enticing walks, I would spend some time reading erotic stories or ogling pictures of naked men. Sometimes I caressed myself lovingly and complimented myself on my beauty, smooth skin, sexy looks, and expert lovemaking technique. As if by magic, the ratio of interested men on the street increased. Guys in the office started making advances. I had more and more dates.

I knew I would eventually have to face the ultimate question. After I went to bed with one of these men, would he find me even more exciting? Or would he discover that my sexy vibes promised something I couldn't deliver?

I had been dating a wonderful man named Michael for several weeks when I knew the big night had arrived. I prepared carefully. Before our date, I flattered and caressed myself. I read my favorite steamy scene from *Lady Chatterley's Lover*. I got out my beefcake pictures and visualized doing all sorts of wicked things to these real-life hunks. I imagined them begging for more and telling me that I was the sexiest creature on two feet.

By the time Michael came to pick me up, I was so excited I could hardly keep my hands off him. But I restrained myself because I wanted to draw things out for the whole evening. I could tell that Michael felt the sexual tension, and I noticed with delight that his tweed trousers seemed to be developing a new bulge. I felt sexier and sexier.

When we finally stepped inside Michael's apartment, we practically ripped the clothes off each other's bodies. I found myself saying and doing things I'd never done before—wonderfully provocative, lusty, lewd things. They just came naturally. And Michael was like a caged animal, panting and circling me, burning with desire. We fondled and kissed each other for hours and then frantically made love in the bed, on the floor, and finally in the shower. Michael said it was the most unbelievable sex of his life; he had never before felt so turned on. And neither had I. My sexual experiment had worked!

That's how I learned the first "Secret of Great Sex."

secret # *1* :

Feel sexy and you will *be* sexy.

No kidding. Try it and see. Many great philosophers have said that you are what you think you are. And it certainly holds true for sexiness. Even if you're not gorgeous, or slender, or voluptuous—even if you're not feeling particularly sexy at the moment. Just conjure up your own sexy self-image. Pretty soon you'll *feel* sexy and therefore *be* sexy. Send out warm, sensuous vibes a man can't help but pick up and he won't even realize you're a little too short or too broad or too fat or too skinny; he'll see you as his own personal sex goddess. And in your sexy mood, you'll just *naturally* do and say wonderfully titillating things. Your touch will be electric. Just the way you glance at his derriere will make his temperature—and other things—rise.

Great sex does not begin with your body or your vagina. *Great sex begins in your head!*

In the following chapters, I will share with you many specific physical techniques for driving a man wild in bed, but they can be truly effective only if you first lay the groundwork by creating a sexy new you. That's what these five secrets of great sex are all about—making yourself into an irresistible sex goddess.

secret #2:

Radiate sexual confidence.

Closely related to Secret #1, the second rule of great sex also springs from a positive and sexy self-image. Again it begins *in your head*.

Usually, the most attractive thing about a person is

his or her self-confidence. Even a beautiful woman will not be more than fleetingly attractive to a man if she is afraid to talk to him, can't meet his eyes, or slouches along embarrassed by or frightened of her own assets. Her actions and words are clear signals that she isn't worth knowing—because *she* doesn't think she is. But a confident woman—even if she has, heaven forbid, *faults*—is magnetically attractive to everyone.

Whenever I ask a man to recall the one trait that made the sexiest woman he ever knew so alluring, invariably he tells me it was her self-confidence. "She carried herself with such assurance." "Liz knew she was hot and you could see it in every move she made." "It's so refreshing not to have to overcome a woman's fears and self-doubts." "Chris is not conventionally beautiful, but sexual electricity crackles all around her. Her self-confidence is very erotic."

So forget about that extra inch of cushioning around your hips. If you think your breasts are too small, try feeling proud of them because they're oh so sensitive to the touch or because your nipples are provocatively pink. I once told a lover that I thought my breasts were too small and I was considering breast enlargement surgery. He immediately cried out, "You mean those sexy, cute little titties that light on fire so good? Oh no! Please leave them the way they are!" And then he hurried me home so he could suck on them for the next two hours. Now I know that the way my sexy little tits "light on fire so good" is one of the greatest turn-ons I can offer a man; and I'm proud and happy to let him enjoy this tasty pleasure.

Get to know and love every inch of your body and mind for the unforgettably sexy woman they make up. If you believe you are the answer to a man's erotic dreams, he'll believe it, too. If you carry yourself with confidence, knowing you're the most interesting and alluring vamp in town, men will be drawn to you like a magnet. And once you're between the sheets, if you are secure in the knowledge that you can drive him really wild in bed, you will!

secret #3:

Concentrate on *him.*

Women who make sex their profession know the surest and most direct way to a man's libido. They focus their attention completely on him, and *only* him. So take a tip from the pros.

Forget about the disagreement you had with the boss earlier. Don't waste time and energy worrying whether your hair looks effectively mussed—or whether your hand isn't better off on his knee than on his elbow. Focus your attention on *him:* his manly chest, his adorable derriere, his playful penis. Make him feel that no one else exists for you but him. No one could possibly be a better, more exciting lover than he is. Let him see that he has truly swept you away with desire.

When you forget yourself and start concentrating instead on your man, you'll find yourself automatically doing wonderfully provocative things to him. They will come naturally to you because of your heightened sexual awareness. You'll do just the things that excite him, not because you have to or because you've painstakingly selected them from your mental bag of sex tricks, but because you just *want* to.

Forget about your own pleasure and focus only on his. What can you do to make him feel wanted? Relaxed? Sexy? Soothed? Ecstatic? As if you can't get enough of him? Fondle him. Caress him. Kiss him lavishly. Lick and nibble him all over. Tell him he's handsome. Strong. Hard. Irresistible. Sexy. A wonderful lover. That he's driving you wild with desire. And mean it! Abandon yourself totally to the joyful task of giving him pleasure; you'll find yourself getting more out of it than he does!

Observe his responses very carefully so you can give him even more of what he *really* likes. Every man has his own personal hot spots and turn-ons. Find out what his are and play on them. Learn to read his pleasure barometer so you'll know what to do more of. Your man may pant when he becomes very excited. His stomach muscles may become tighter, his testicles harder, or his nipples more pronounced. Maybe he moans and groans, or shudders, or starts thrusting convulsively.

Get to know your man's personal preferences so you can play him like a finely tuned instrument. The music you make will give both of you extraordinary pleasure. And your man will find that, for some reason, no one knows how to make him feel quite as good as you do. He just can't help coming back for more. And the more you give, the more you'll *get*.

secret #4:

Do unto him what he does unto you.

Make mental notes of the special places he touches you and the way he does it; then later do the same to him. If he plants light butterfly kisses on your eyelids, you should do the same for him. If he twirls your nipples slowly between thumb and forefinger, he probably has sensitive nipples himself and would welcome your reciprocal nipple massage. Without realizing it, your man is telling you exactly what he likes in bed by doing it to you first; it's a subconscious urge we all have. And you can use it to great advantage.

Don't mimic his moves right away. Wait until the next time you make love—and then "surprise" him with your intimate knowledge of his personal sexual preferences. As if by magic, or with some sexy sixth sense, you'll be reading his mind and body—doing exactly what drives him to the heights of ecstasy. How do you know him so well?

secret # 5 :

See your sexuality as a sacred gift.

Your sexuality is unique to you. No one else has a sexual nature quite like yours. No other woman expresses her passion just the way you do. No one else possesses quite the same wonderful blend of giving and receiving, soft and hard, yielding and rough, as you do.

The feel of your skin, the sound of your moans, the curve of your neck, the look of passion in your eyes, the smell of your excitement—all these things are uniquely yours. No other woman looks, feels, sounds, smells, or tastes quite like you do. None moves like you do. None responds to a lover's touch in quite the same way. No other woman writhes in ecstasy when her man licks her little toe. No other woman has a rough spot on her tongue that tickles his nipple so maddeningly. No other woman magically turns into satin at the briefest touch of his hand.

Your sexuality is unique because *you* are unique. It is your one-of-a-kind expression of the basic life force, the energy that creates new life. It is one of the most powerful, enduring, and creative forces on earth. This tremendous power is yours to command, to enjoy, and to give as a very special and sacred gift. When you value yourself and the gift of your sexuality in this way, it becomes even more radiant and exciting. You take on a luminous and tantalizing glow that literally gives off sparks.

And when you cherish your lover's unique sexuality as well, he will feel like an adored king. How could he resist the woman who makes him feel like the sexiest, most desirable creature on earth? The woman who treats him like an endless treasure house of delights? With you, he feels like the acme of male sexual power; a magical potentate capable of creating, and worthy of receiving, unknown ecstasies; a sex god playing with a luscious sex goddess. Powerful stuff!

These five "Secrets of Great Sex" form the cornerstone on which you can build a truly great sexual life. Without them, even the most exotic tricks will seem merely mechanical and possibly even insulting. But with these secrets firmly established as a base, even the simplest gesture will take on highly erotic overtones. So remember them well!

s e c r e t # 1 :

Feel sexy and you will *be* sexy.

s e c r e t # 2 :

Radiate sexual confidence.

secret **#3:**

Concentrate on *him*.

secret **#4:**

Do unto him what he does unto you.

secret **#5:**

See your sexuality as a sacred gift.

Great sex begins in the mind. If you create sexiness and passion in your head, you'll soon find the real thing in your bed. In no time, you'll be inventing your own special ways to drive your man wild in bed. But just to get you started, here are 203 tested man pleasers.

i like my body when it is

with your / body. It is so

quite new a thing. /

Muscles better and nerves

more . . . / And eyes big

love-crumbs, / and possibly

i like the thrill / of under

me you so quite new

—E. E. Cummings

2

setting
the
stage

$g$reat sex doesn't happen by itself. It takes preparation and practice. It takes getting to know and like your body, finding out what it can do, and strengthening the muscles you will be using. It means developing confidence in yourself and your body.

So if you are unhappy with the general condition of your body, do something about it. But remember, it's not necessary to be physically perfect (no one is!) to have great sex. It *is* necessary, however, for you to get comfortable with your body — and tone up your sensual nerve endings and your sex muscles because they have a direct bearing on the level of passion you and your man will reach. Far from being an arduous and boring task, this sexual toning-up is a titillating experience all by itself. So, let's get started.

getting to
know yourself

One of the greatest turn-ons for a man is to see how very much he's exciting you; he wants to know that his lovemaking is driving *you* wild in bed. The only way to arrange it so he stimulates you, and therefore himself, to the max (what a delicious assignment!) is for you to know beforehand where all your sexual switches are and how they are turned on. The ancient wisdom applies here: Know thyself. If you aren't already familiar with your own body, take the time to start getting acquainted right now.

Remove all your clothes and stand in front of a mirror. Investigate every square inch of your body. Don't be judgmental; your objective is self-knowledge, not self-criticism. Note the sensuous slope of your breasts. Mark the difference between the two. Delight in the pinkness or brownness of your nipples. Really look at the curve of your waist and hips, the swell of your abdomen, the strength of your legs. Arrange another mirror so you can get a good view of your languorous back and fetching fanny. Inspect everything as if you were going to do a detailed drawing of your naked body from memory. Imagine every part in action. Imagine every part from a man's point of view.

Then see what happens when you touch yourself.

Run your hands over your silky skin. Blow on it. Rub a rough cloth against it. Tickle yourself with a feather. Lick the places you can reach. Scrape your nails lightly across the surface. Massage, knead, and caress yourself all over. Cover *every* inch. Find out what feels best, most relaxing, most exciting.

Fondle your breasts. Massage them in circles with the flat of your palm. Pull on the nipples. Twirl them between your fingers. Wet your fingers and touch them to your nipples. Rub them with something rough, smooth, hard, soft, cold, hot. Watch them become erect and hard. Observe the sway and jiggle of your breasts. They may become flushed. They may develop goose-flesh. Imagine how a man would react to the feel and look of them. What would you want him to do with them? Try it yourself. Roam over your entire body in this fashion, observing and feeling everything that happens, imagining how a man would see it, feel about it, react to it.

Squat over a mirror and inspect your genitalia. Spread apart the outer lips; notice their color and shape, feel their texture. Scrutinize your clitoris, urethra, and vaginal opening; notice their size and relative positions. Feel their smoothness, their bumps and valleys, the ridginess of the outer vaginal rim. Slowly insert a clean forefinger into your vagina, circling to touch all surfaces, reaching the rough end of the passageway at the cervix. Marvel at its moist warmth. Squeeze your finger with your vaginal muscles and see how it feels. Know that a man's penis enjoys this same sucking feeling.

Remove your finger and massage your entire genital area with it. Move up to the clitoris and circle it gently. Use one finger, three fingers, your whole hand. Press firmly, gently, insistently, languorously, slowly, then faster. Does it become larger? Deeper in color? Do juices flow from your vagina? How does it feel to insert a finger into your vagina at the same time you are massaging your clitoris? To thrust the finger in and out? What can you dream up to make it feel even better?

Besides being immensely pleasurable, masturbation keeps your sex muscles in shape and is the best way to find out what really turns you on. Once you know your own sexual preferences, you can show your man how to satisfy them. Nothing turns a guy on more than watching and feeling a lovely woman writhe with sexual pleasure under his fingers and tongue. So be creative and adventurous when you masturbate; explore all the possibilities of your libido. You may come upon a teeth-chattering climax—and what fun to show your man how to do it for you! Here are some ideas to get you started on the creative exploration of your erogenous zones:

- Watch yourself in the mirror. Be sure you can see *everything.*

- Thrust a dildo or any penis-like object in and out of your vulva; a cucumber, a candle, a carrot or zucchini, a small plastic bottle, or whatever. Don't use anything sharp or breakable, especially not an open bottle, as it will form suction and you won't be able to remove it.

- Massage your clitoris with a vibrator and slide it around the entire vaginal area. Insert it into your vagina. A vibrator can also be great for tingling the nipples.

- It's not easy, but if you can position your clitoris under the falling water from the bathtub faucet, you'll enjoy a very erotic sensation. If you have a movable shower massage, you can be very versatile with your watery sexercises.

- While you are pleasuring your genitals, don't forget to play with your breasts, too. Most women's nipples are directly connected to their sex organs. Pull on your nipples, twirl them between your fingers, rub them with a rough cloth or object. This will increase the sensation in your genital area.

- Excite yourself by looking at sexy pictures of men or women, or both. Read erotic literature. Talk dirty to yourself or to an imaginary bed partner. Find out what you like best.

- Insert ice cubes into your vagina. Or cherries, grapes, mashed bananas, orange sections. Use your erotic imagination.

The more you learn about your sexual appetites and desires, the more you can teach your man about pleasing you—which in turn pleases him. And the more you pleasure yourself, the sexier you'll feel; all the better to entice him into your bed.

Your man's penis gets very excited when it slips inside your moist, warm vagina; and the friction created by moving in and out intensifies the sensation. But far more than just a receptacle for your man's "sword of love," your vagina is a versatile and sensual sheath with active abilities of its own. You can give him an almost unbearably delicious thrill by learning to flex your sex muscle. By that I mean your pubococcygeus, or PC muscle. This is the muscle that allows you to stop the flow of your urine; the same one that contracts when you have an orgasm. The twitching of the PC muscle against your man's penis is a wonderfully erotic and highly stimulating sensation for both of you. Try inserting three fingers into your vagina and flexing that muscle. See what I mean? As with any other muscle, the PC muscle gets stronger with use. To develop a superbly sexy vagina, practice contracting your PC muscle at least twenty-five times every day. Soon you'll have an exquisitely toned man pleaser.

Here's another great vaginal exercise. Place a dildo, vibrator, candle, cucumber, or the like inside your vagina. Sitting straight up and using only your developing sex muscle, try to keep it there. Don't let it slip out. See if you can walk around while still holding the object in place. Now lie down and try to push it out. Practice until you can squirt it out forcefully. First you keep it locked inside, then you send it flying. Just think what you'll be able to do to him!

Now that you're all sexy and ready to go, let's get started on your man! The first of 203 ways to drive him wild in or out of bed is yours when you read on.

mental foreplay

Your brain is the most erotic part of your body. Always remember that it's what goes on in your head that sets the tone, makes you feel and act sexy, and conjures up all the deliciously erotic things you're going to do. You know how aroused you become when thinking about stroking your man's chest or his taut derriere, or how he sucked your nipples the last time you were together, or the way Richard Gere kissed Debra Winger in *An Officer and a Gentleman*. Well, he gets just as turned on thinking about your lovely, warm vagina, or the way you licked his ear last night, or what happened in the blue movie he saw last Tuesday. Imagination is the sexiest turn-on of all. So if you want to be an expert lover, you should learn and practice the fine art of mental foreplay. Give him something to think about that will make him hot and bothered, something that will make him crazy to get his hands on you, something that will make him deliciously hard. Sex up his imagination and you'll reap the erotic rewards.

1. Tell him about the self-massage, internal flexing, and voyeuristic activities you've been doing to get ready for him. Give him every luscious detail. Invite him to watch.

2. Show him "dirty" pictures. The surest turn-ons are those of women making love to each other or explicit shots of a man and a woman having sex. These are easy to come by in the "men's entertainment" magazines—or in wonderfully erotic books like Helmut Newton's *Sleepless Nights* (men find this irresistible), *Japanese Nights* (reproductions of erotic prints), *The Erotic Drawings of Fragonard* (elegant and lascivious eighteenth-century French lovers), and books showing those amazing Indian temple sculptures in their contorted but very sexy positions. You can say you saw something interesting you'd like his opinion on.

3. Show him erotic pictures of *you*. Have a girlfriend

take them (you can do the same for her) and surprise him with your centerfold beauty.

4. Mail him an explicit nude photo of yourself—no note, no return address, just kiss the back of the envelope with your signature lip color and let it be from naughty you.

5. Ask *him* to take pictures of you. Pretend that you're posing for *Playboy* or *Penthouse*. Act like a sex kitten.

6. Use a camera with a timer to take snapshots of the two of you *together;* you massaging his erection, him licking your nipples, the two of you savoring one of your favorite lovemaking positions.

7. Read him some erotic literature. But don't use the romantic stuff. He'll want to hear something very racy. Try *A Man with a Maid* by Anonymous, *Plaisir d'Amour* by Anne-Marie Villefranche, *The Delta of Venus* by Anaïs Nin, *The Pearl* (collected Victorian erotica), any of the Black Cat paperbacks, or any of the erotic stories in *Playboy* or *Penthouse*.

$8.$ Tape-record your lovemaking session. Then play it back when you want to arouse him the second—or third—time. Or have it spliced into the middle of the Ravel's *Bolero* tape you like to put on at romantic moments. He'll be warmly surprised!

$9.$ Write him a lewd note and slip it secretly into his jacket or pants pocket, or tuck it into his *Wall Street Journal.*

$10.$ Rent some porno videos and have a private screening. Some classics to try are *Deep Throat, Illusions of a Lady* (more artistic than most), and *The Green Door.*

$11.$ The telephone can be a very sexy instrument. Give him an unexpected call—at work, or when one of you is out of town—and tell him you're going to spend all night sucking his nipples, then his navel, then his luscious bottom, and then his gorgeous penis; or he's the sexiest man you've ever known and you can't wait to feel him inside you; or you're lying in bed nude and pretending he's biting you here, fingering you there, kissing you everywhere, and it feels *so* good (add some heavy breathing and moaning). Go into juicy detail, and then hang up quickly. The sexual suspense will keep him hot for hours.

 1 2. Another way to use some sexy talk as a mental warm-up is to save it up for an occasion when you're out together in public; in a restaurant, at a formal party, waiting in line for the movies, at a concert, whenever. Look him straight in the eye and, in a completely normal voice so no one would guess what you're saying, tell him what you intend to do to him later. Be very specific. Then smile sweetly and adroitly change the subject. Be sure to fulfill your promises later.

 1 3. Suggest that he buy you the sexiest piece of lingerie or leather he can find. You might give him a Victoria's Secret or a Frederick's of Hollywood catalog to browse through. When the item he orders arrives, model it for him and put yourself at his disposal for the evening.

 1 4. Tell him that you're going to buy him some underwear with a hole cut out for his special equipment and that when he wears it, you're going to do some very erotic things to him. Then do it.

 1 5. Send him some erotic underwear in the mail. Include a note about how you plan to use it.

$16.$ Take him to the opera in your formal clothes and confide in him that you "forgot" to wear your panties, so you have nothing on underneath. Let him think about that all evening.

$17.$ Arrange for a flower to be delivered to him, but make it an erotic one: a *Paphiopedilum* orchid, a bird of paradise, a brilliant tiger lily. Include a sexy note.

$18.$ One of the most devastating sexual weapons you have is the odor of your vaginal juices. Men may joke about the smell of fish, but if you keep yourself clean, the musky perfume of your natural lubricant can make an incredible aphrodisiac. The odor of a female "in heat" is meant to attract the male of the species; so use it. Before you see your man, use some of your own *cassolette* as you would your favorite perfume: a touch behind the ears, at the throat, between your breasts, on your wrists. He'll wonder why he can't keep his hands—and his mouth—off you.

$19.$ Speaking of aphrodisiacs, try the powerful magic of aromatherapy to entice and excite your lover. Using essential oils as a perfume for you, the room, or the bath is an ancient and still quite potent way to weave the web of seduction. Cleopatra did this expertly. So can you. Sensual fragrances like rose (the queen of feminine scents), jasmine (the king of masculine scents), ylang-ylang, sandalwood, patchouli, white ginger, and musk are sure to warm the cockles of his erogenous zones.

20. Share one of your fantasies. Even the idea that you *have* fantasies will be titillating to him; it shows you're a woman who enjoys thinking about sex and who has an erotic imagination. Tell him all the juicy details and, if appropriate, suggest you act them out. You might want to start with one of your tamer fantasies and, depending on his response, move on to the kinkier ones.

21. Ask him to share his fantasies with you. Listen attentively and don't be shocked at anything he says or you'll frighten him off. Sharing each other's fantasies is a terribly intimate, revealing, and erotic act. So be tender and understanding when he bares his sexual soul to you. Then tell him how much his fantasy turns you on and ask if he minds acting it out with you. Unless he's painfully inhibited, he'll be thrilled you want his dream to come true.

making a love nest

The surroundings in which your lovemaking occurs are almost as important as the lovemaking itself. Drab or boring digs can make for drab, boring sex; while sensuous, provocative, or new locations set the stage for heightened sexual experience. French courtesans during the reign of Louis XIV, the Sun King, took great care to create a very special, sensuous environment for their trysts with the nobility. They would sometimes completely redecorate for each different man, including special bedsheets with a design and scent known to please a particular lover. They carefully considered how to stimulate *each* of a man's senses—beautiful environs with erotic pictures or statues for the eye; sensuous and soothing music for the ear; evocative scents and pungent perfumes for the nose; luscious, juicy fruits and wines to taste; rich, voluptuous fabrics and surfaces to touch. They surrounded their paramours with an aura of irresistible sensuality that brought out each man's sexual best.

Take a cue from these great sexual gourmets and open a whole new world of erotic pleasure for yourself and your man. Remember that the surroundings you create must be those that will arouse *his* senses, not necessarily just yours. This takes some observation and careful thought. Watch closely for the things he responds to and then duplicate or enhance them in your lovemaking environment.

In the section on Mental Foreplay, we talked about some immediate ways to excite your man with sexy sights and sounds. Here are some ideas for creating a constant undercurrent of sensuality in your surroundings.

$22.$ Place erotic Japanese prints, elegant, sexy photos, and sensuous statuettes in strategic locations in your bedroom, then draw his attention to them at crucial moments. Maybe *that* position would be fun.

$23.$ Indulge in flora: lots of plants in the bedroom may make a man feel like he's in the jungle and, if so, they should bring out his more primitive instincts. Cut flowers will create an aura of refined romance that will please both the eyes and the nose. And flower petals are so lovely for tickling each other.

$24.$ A fur throw or a thick, soft rug is very sensuous to naked bodies. All fabrics in the bedroom should invite the touch; soft cotton, smooth silk or satin, rich velvet, deep pile rugs, overstuffed chairs, fluffy pillows, cozy comforters, or nubby bedspreads. All these sensations will invite his touch on your silky skin.

$25.$ Play sensuous background music. Find out whether his taste runs to dreamy ballads, classical, soft rock, or maybe the sounds of the ocean, and make a continuous tape you can put on and leave for a while. After that, focus your attention on him, not the music.

$26.$ Scent the room or the sheets *lightly* with a musky or flowery perfume, depending upon his preference. Everything else should smell fresh and clean. Once he begins to associate that particular scent with your lovemaking, you can start using it judiciously at other times and places. It'll put him in the mood immediately.

$27.$ Always have some chilled wine ready for before-, during-, and after-sex sipping. Fresh fruit is a refreshing appetizer for the next sexual course and can become a play toy as well (more about that in chapter 3). For an occasional treat, prepare a bed picnic. Use only finger foods. You'll know what to prepare if you think of that famous food foreplay scene in the movie *Tom Jones.* Don't forget napkins!

$28.$ Lighting is crucial! Get rid of any bright, glaring lamps, but—and this is important—leave enough light for him to see how sexy you look and to watch the two of you perform one of the most visually exciting acts known to man or woman. A man delights in seeing your face flush with excitement, your breasts sway to his rhythm, your hips writhe, and his penis disappearing inside your sexy vagina. So don't deprive him of his visual turn-ons, and yours, too.

But keep the lighting soft. Candles are really the best choice (large, simple ones are preferred, scented if you like), but you can achieve some lovely effects by changing one light bulb to red, pink, or even green or blue. Then use only that lamp and perhaps a candle or two.

29. If you can manage it, it's marvelous to have a mirrored wall or a very large mirror beside, in front of, or above the bed. Watching the reflection of your own lovemaking can't be beat as an exciting natural turn-on.

30. Your bed should be large enough to roll around in, strong and silent enough to withstand some fairly energetic activities, and soft enough to be languidly comfortable for hours. Never bring a man to a messy, unmade bed, and always make sure the sheets are fresh and clean. Lots of pillows and soft blankets or comforters are extremely sensuous. Soft pure cotton sheets are the best and most comfortable, but you may want to try satin sheets for "special" occasions. Every-

thing about the bed should make your man feel completely comfortable and slightly spoiled.

3 1 . Next to the bed you should keep a small stack of all the sexual necessities: condoms, lubricants, creams and body oils, a small clean towel, tissues, your diaphragm or whatever method of birth control you use, erotic literature and pictures, and any sexual toys and props you like to play with (vibrators, feathers, silk cords, dildos, beads, what have you). If you are prepared, you won't have to leave in the middle of something interesting.

3 2 . One of the most flattering things you can do for a man is to change or add to the sexual ambience after you've learned what his preferences are. When you discover he loves black, get some black velvet throw pillows for your boudoir. Grapes are his favorite fruit? Bring some to bed. He's into feathers? Stock up on all sizes, shapes, and textures. This kind of stroke to his sexual ego should spur him on to new heights of passion.

adventuring out of the nest

Now that you've made your bedroom into a sensuous haven, it's time to start branching out. Sex in the same place, and at the same predictable time, quickly becomes routine and dull. A truly erotic playmate will add spice to a long-term love affair by initiating sex in varied and unusual places, and at unexpected times. Something as simple as moving to a different room can lend an air of special excitement to your sex play. Men love variety, and you can provide all the novelty he'll ever need by being creative about where you seduce him. You can organize an outing to some untried or exotic spot—or simply have a spontaneous sex tryst in a corner where you are in danger of being discovered at any moment.

The thrill of unexpected or "dangerous" sex is a big turn-on and worth every effort or inconvenience it may cause. Remember Burt Lancaster and Deborah Kerr rolling in the surf in *From Here to Eternity?* The erotic sex in an empty apartment from *Last Tango in Paris?* The under-the-table activities of Julie Christie in *Shampoo*?

These are the kinds of highly charged moments that aren't too difficult to create and that, once experienced, will be etched in your man's erotic memory forever.

$33.$ One of the simplest changes of scenery you can make is to move your lovemaking to another room. Seduce him unexpectedly while you're both watching TV in the den. That big armchair would make a marvelous playpen. Later you can slide onto the rug. How about the extra bedroom? The living room? The dining room table? The bathroom—on the john or on the floor? Try the kitchen counter; or just stand up against the refrigerator. The attic can be wickedly nostalgic, and the basement excitingly bizarre. Or try the study for intellectually stimulating sex. The stairs are great for interesting positions. The closet *under* the stairs is wonderfully furtive. The front vestibule. Your dressing room. All are incredibly erotic spots for love trysts, if you make them so.

$34.$ Move outside. How pleasantly surprised he'll be when you "attack" him in your very own bushes. Make love on the back-porch swing. Seduce him in the hammock, or by moonlight in the garden. If you live in an apartment, you might have to be a little more inventive to enjoy backyard sex, but the thrill of possible discovery will add extra spice to your mating. If you can get onto the roof of your building, take advantage of this starlit setting for love.

$35.$ While not exactly out*doors*, the elevator is out-

side your apartment, and can you think of anything naughtier than holding the DOOR CLOSE button against intruders while you pound into each other, standing against the elevator wall?

36. Don't forget about your own portable cocoon, the car. Making love to you in the backseat will make him feel as potent and horny as he did in high school; and lucky you will be on the receiving end of his reborn virility.

37. Surprise him at the office. Bring a picnic lunch, ask his secretary to hold all calls, close the door, and treat him to a desktop delight. If you're really daring, you can try a quickie in the office elevator; but don't get caught by his boss!

38. Parties are made for excitingly "dangerous" sex. Tease him all evening with your sultry eyes and secretly roving hands. Then slip into your host's bathroom, bedroom, or closet and culminate the act. You might even want to leave the door ajar and hide behind it. If it's an outdoor party, all the better. Sneak off to the bushes, behind a sand dune, or the nearest big tree, where the murmur of the party crowd can serve as your background music.

39. Ask him to meet you at a hotel for drinks. Then either meet him in the lobby and take him up to the room you've rented to show him a "surprise," or leave a message for him to go to a specific room. When he walks in, he'll find you with little on your body and a lot of sex on your mind.

40. Take him for a drive in the country and stop in some secluded spot to admire the view. Then create your own "splendor in the grass."

41. Arrange to borrow a friend's apartment or house while he or she is out. Then tell your man you want to take him there and make love to him mercilessly. The idea of having sex in somebody else's bed, or on somebody's else's floor or couch, will start his mind and his pulse racing. You might try this out with the apartment of your friend, the local Casanova. I think you'll find your man taking on some of this great lover's characteristics!

42. On a workday, invite him to your place for lunch. Serve a light meal, a bottle of good wine, and some seductive smiles. Let him discover for himself that you're wearing nothing underneath your terribly busi-

nesslike suit. After an exciting tumble in bed, you'll both be much better prepared to tackle the rest of the work-day.

43. Get him to the beach and re-create the surf-sex scene in *From Here to Eternity*. Or go skinny-dipping in the moonlight and caress him underwater. You can float into some wonderfully exotic positions with ease or just enjoy the extremely sensual rocking and sliding sensations the water gives you. This one makes for erotic fireworks!

44. Reserve a private room with hot tub at your health club. Once there, you should become your man's personal masseuse and give him a very thorough rub-down. You can't do this properly unless you're both nude, although you are allowed to drape a towel over the parts of his body you're not working on. That's so he won't get cold. Depending on the mood of the moment, you may want to delay any serious sexual overtures un-til after the two of you emerge from a long soak in the tub—and you're both good and hot. Lick him dry and carry on from there. He won't soon forget this steamy, dreamy interlude!

45. Okay, you've heard about it and probably

thought it impossible, but yes, you *can* have sex in an airplane bathroom; and it's a wonderfully elevating experience. Actually, the trickiest part is getting in and out of the cubicle unnoticed by the line of people waiting to use it. So try to take your mile-high spin during the movie, while they're serving a meal, or at some other low bathroom-occupancy period.

Once you've rendezvoused in the bathroom, the easiest position to achieve is probably him seated on the toilet (lid closed) and you seated on his lap, facing in either direction. Both of you standing works too, if your heights are sexually compatible. Of course, hand and/or tongue massages are also possible and are equally exhilarating. Whichever method you choose, it's an excellent way to relieve the boredom of a long flight!

games and toys

When you're in a playful mood, or want to break the ice after a period of abstinence, or you sense the need for yet another kind of variety, there's nothing like a good old erotic game or sex toy. The Japanese have been playing with sex toys for centuries and have developed the art of erotic gamesmanship to a high degree.

A geisha girl's main purpose in life was to pleasure a man in the most elegant and ingenious way possible. So her sexual bag of tricks was chock-full of fascinating props and titillating head games. Many of the gadgets

you'll find in your local sex paraphernalia store origi-
nated with those clever Asians and are well worth a test
spin.

Become familiar with all the merchandise in the store
so you can pick and choose what's right for you. If you
can't imagine what that weird contraption in the corner
is for, don't be afraid to ask the salesperson. He's heard
it all before, at least twice, and it won't even occur to
him to think of you as anything but another nice cus-
tomer. You're sure to find at least one thing that will
pique your curiosity. Take it home and see how many
ways you and your man can divine for using this fascinating toy.

Challenge him to a game of strip poker, crazy eights,
or even chess. Dream up a playful scenario for the two
of you to act out. Many of the most exciting sex games
don't need props at all—only your wonderfully lascivious mind. Your erotic imagination will set the only lim-
itation on the number and variety of lusty diversions
you can invent. Try anything and everything you can
think of. Men love adventure.

46. Use your vibrator on him. Or purchase a different kind for his pleasure only. Massage him with the
Swedish type that fits on top of your hand. This provides the gentlest stimulation but still gives quite a marvelous tingle to the penis and testicles.

Experiment with the various attachments on your

regular vibrator. See what works best on his nipples, penis, scrotum, anus, and the sensitive spot between. Always use the other hand to maintain the warm contact of flesh against flesh; otherwise he may feel a little too "mechanized." Don't press too hard, and make very sensuous, smooth, slow movements. Treat the vibrator like an intensely stimulating version of your hand — which it is. Caress all his favorite hot spots.

47. If you have a very self-assured and open-minded man, you may find he'll enjoy receiving the attentions of your vibrating dildo. Use it like a regular vibrator or, with a little lubrication and a lot of patience, you can even try massaging his anus with it. As long as he doesn't see it as an affront to his masculinity, both of you can enjoy the marvelous sensation of you "having a penis" for a change.

48. Your local sex shop should have a large variety of ticklers. These are little sleeves that fit over the end of the penis and come equipped with bumps, soft prongs, ridges, and other little goodies designed to stimulate your vagina. Buy a few and invite your man to "tickle" you.

49. Another gadget for your man's penis is a cock

ring, a small rubber or metal doughnut that fits snugly around the base of his penis. Some are meant to fit around his testicles, too. Others are straps of leather with snaps at the end. A cock ring helps to keep him really hard and feeling pleasantly swollen and huge. He'll feel and act as if he's playing a Stradivarius instead of his everyday "instrument."

50. Buy a set of erotic cards — or make your own. The action cards should say things like "kiss," "suck," "lick," "bite." The body cards name various parts: "ear," "nipple," "toe," "penis," and so on. Take turns picking a card from each pile and applying the instructions to your partner for five minutes a turn.

51. Ask him to tie you to the bed and take his pleasure of you.

52. Tie him to the bed and ravish him mercilessly.

53. Challenge him to a duel; the first one to "shoot" (have an orgasm) loses. The winner gets treated to an erotic evening of his or her choice. Enjoy the struggle!

54. Play strip backgammon, strip Trivial Pursuit, or strip cribbage. Of course, there's always black jack, hearts, dominoes, Scrabble, or whatever. You name it, you can strip to it.

55. Speaking of stripping, practice your striptease artistry and perform for him. Use veils, feathers, gloves, garter belts, whatever you can think of, and toss them provocatively in his direction. Throw in lots of bumps and grinds to the rhythm of the music. You may want to close the show by caressing your freshly revealed breasts, stomach, and bushy triangle, and inviting him to join you.

56. Call him at work with the trivia question for the day. Explain that if he answers correctly, you'll be his sex slave for two hours that evening. If he doesn't get the right answer, *he* must be *your* sex slave. Make the question moderately difficult so that he'll feel truly challenged; and if he doesn't get it, give him another chance the next day and then the next, till he finally succeeds in winning you for a luscious slave.

57. On a lazy Sunday when you'll be staying in all

day, demand that he remain in the nude for the duration. Tease him with playful caresses and love slaps all day, then pay it off that night.

58. Reverse these roles and parade around naked all day. Tell him to use you as he will.

59. Play erotic charades. The rules of the game are these: (1) Both players must be nude. (2) One partner acts out the sexual activity he or she wants to do. For instance, if you point to your man, then lick your lips, squeeze your nipples, and finally hold up the fingers of both hands, he may correctly guess that you want him to lick your nipples for ten minutes. (3) No matter how provocative these charades may look, you cannot touch each other until the charade is solved correctly. (4) When the correct answer is given, your partner wins the privilege of performing the act in question. (5) Reverse your roles for the next charade. (6) Continue the game until you get too involved to notice.

60. "Name That Flavor" is a lovely game, too. Anoint your vulva with flavored extract of love oil and make him guess what it is by licking it off. Turn about is fair play, and he must have his chance at

stumping you by dabbing a mystery flavor on his penis and letting your tongue perform its investigations. No further love play is allowed until the licker names that flavor, or until the lickee can't stand it anymore.

"A lady always behaves

in a manner appropriate to

the occasion. The proper

behavior for foreplay is

unbridled passion,

tenderness, eagerness to

please, admiration, humor,

and love. No wonder the

uninhibited lady is a

lovable lady!"

—*"J," Total Loving*

3
fabulous
foreplay

Most men are very nervous about foreplay. They vaguely understand that they don't spend enough time with it but are uncertain as to how to remedy the situation. Most men simply don't realize that foreplay can be at least as exciting and satisfying as intercourse— sometimes more so. The poor darlings haven't learned how to relax and enjoy the anticipation, the mounting tension, the electricity of hot skin against hotter skin, the magic of a suddenly juicy vagina, the glorious swelling of his own organ. Only a woman—a very sensitive, sensuous woman—can show a man how to truly enjoy the splendor of good foreplay. And only you can show your man what a rapturous experience he can have when you come alive under his hands and slowly and deliciously get him hotter and harder than he's ever been.

I learned just how true this is when I was traveling abroad some years ago. In one Mediterranean country, the men are very handsome and supposedly very hot in bed. But they are too concerned with how many positions they can get into and how hard they can pump in and out. This can be very invigorating, but ultimately less than totally satisfying. The women of this country admit to being very submissive in the sack and wouldn't think of suggesting a different pattern of lovemaking. So the men go on with their uninspired shoving and pawing, and neither men nor women get to experience the joy of fine lovemaking to its fullest.

When I began a luscious affair with one of these men, I decided to try initiating him into these finer pleasures. At first, I worried that his sense of macho would suffer, and in fact it will if you're not sensitive about it. But with careful handling, I found this marvelous man to be more than a willing pupil and a very fast and eager learner. Once he discovered what deliciously languorous sensations he'd been missing, he learned to savor a nice long session of hot foreplay. He discovered that a sweet, slow buildup can make the final event so much more powerful. And I, of course, reaped the splendid rewards. We were both vastly enriched.

So don't deprive your man of truly exquisite sex. Show him what fine foreplay is all about, because he probably won't have a clue. Once he gets a taste, he'll develop an addiction.

When introducing your man to the wonders of foreplay "à la you," keep three things in mind:

1. *Think sexy.*
2. *Think inventive.*
3. *Think relaxed.*

Think sexy because that's the basic rule of great love-making. And it's very important here because the whole idea is for both of you to feel sexier longer.

Think inventive because that's what makes foreplay exciting enough for him to be jolted out of his old lovemaking patterns. Give him something different, something succulent, something a little kinky, something that will get him very hot and bothered.

Think relaxed because you need to establish a mood of leisurely, sustained passion. If you can get him to sit back, relax, and enjoy the buildup, you've got him hooked, and you're both in for a treat.

Of course, foreplay overlaps with all the other stages of lovemaking. It doesn't always come first, and it may be an end unto itself. So you'll find suggestions here that overlap with areas covered in other chapters of this book and some that you may want to use *after* intercourse or fellatio or someplace else. Be ready to look at these suggestions in a new way. Good foreplay can come in handy anywhere, anytime. After all, foreplay is really anything that makes him hot and hard (or harder), and you hot and juicy (or juicier). Have a ball!

kissing

Kissing is a very fine art. But because we do it so often and for such divergent reasons, sometimes we forget just how erotic a deeply felt or unusually placed kiss can be. Don't. If you approach each kiss with a sense of wonder (you are actually putting your incredibly soft, sensitive lips on his soft, pliant and very personal mouth, and you may even touch tongues!), you'll be well on your way to creating a very sensual experience. Concentrate on the sensation of lip against lip, tongue on tongue, wet against dry, and you'll startle him into an early erection. He too will remember the excitement and electric discovery of a first kiss, the voluptuous magnetism of a pair of ripe, pouty lips. Be inventive. Use your lips, your tongue, your teeth. Press hard. Brush softly. Suck, lick, and bite. Linger lovingly, press passionately. And *respond sensitively* to his lip maneuvers. This is not a solo tune but a lovely, harmonious duet.

61. Lick only the corners of his mouth, two highly erogenous spots.

62. Offer him the inside of your lips while kissing deeply; it's much softer and more sensitive, and it's a deeply intimate gesture.

63. Caress his face, the side of his neck, the back of his head, or hold his head and face between your two hands as you assault his mouth with kisses.

64. Run your tongue over his gums, around his tongue, across his lips; then follow it up with a nibble or a localized kiss.

65. While enjoying some lovely open-mouthed kisses, pause for a while, mouths still open on each other, and simply breathe each other's breath. This is very hot!

66. I know a man who gets very excited when, instead of one extended kiss, I give him many short, sucking kisses, one right after another; he seems to want to reach inside me for more. Try it with your man.

67. Here's a kissing technique from the *Ananga Ranga,* an ancient Indian text on lovemaking similar to the famous *Kama Sutra.* Cover his eyes with your hands and thrust your tongue into his mouth. Move your tongue from side to side and in and out, using motions that suggest more intimate forms of enjoyment to come. Something about the vulnerability and mystery of having his eyes covered enhances this sweet sensation for your lover.

oneplay for two

$68.$ Give him a private show he'll never forget. Masturbate for him. Almost every man dreams of watching a sexy woman play with herself provocatively, but they almost never get to make this dream come true. Most women are too shy for this kind of very hot teasing. But when you see the look of naked desire this behavior produces on your man's face, you'll quickly overcome any inhibitions.

$69.$ Ask him to lick your fingers while you masturbate yourself with them. *Very* hot!

$70.$ Ask him to masturbate for you.

clothing as a prop

$71.$ Wear no undies and, at the appropriate moment, flash him.

72. Give him an erotic surprise by taking off your business suit or casual outfit to reveal a bra with the nipples cut out, a half bra, crotchless panties, or a lacy garter belt over no panties.

73. Take care over your bedwear. Don't forget that the mystery of what's hidden is often more provocative than the naked truth. Sexy items are: a slinky black nightgown (yes, it's a cliché, but it still works!); the virginal look of a pure white cotton nightgown with long sleeves and high neck; men's pajamas, shirt, or underwear; a filmy lace gown, camisole, or teddy; a light silk robe left open in front; anything see-through, as long as it's loose. Then flaunt it!

74. Play dress-up. Costume yourself as a maid, soldier, waitress, nurse, torch singer, another man, circus performer, dairy maid, or whatever his secret erotic wish may be. Dress him up, too, and play out the suggested roles.

75. Undress slowly and seductively. Slide each piece of clothing over your skin as you remove it and hold it in front of you briefly before you let it drop to the floor. Lift your leg and point your toe or prop your leg

prettily on a chair as you push your stockings off. Toss them in your man's direction. Ask him to undo your zipper, then back away. Lift your arms high and arch your back as you remove your shirt; this pushes your breasts up and out. Stretch and arch with catlike grace at every opportunity.

When you get down to your bra and panties, you may want to turn your back to him as you slip off one or the other, then slowly face him with your nakedness. Or let him watch as you glide your hands over your nipples while removing your bra or over your bushy triangle as you drop your panties. Performing this striptease in candlelight will give your body a soft glow and help to camouflage any of your less-than-perfect features.

76. Ask him to undress you. Help him out by stretching languorously as he removes each item.

77. Undress him. Take it slow and easy, and kiss and fondle him as you go. Start with his shirt and slide it sensuously off his back with both hands. It's a nice touch to caress your face with his shirt, taking in his masculine aroma; he'll feel very special. To avoid a hopeless muddle, remove his footwear before going for his pants. Then, in preparation for undoing the zipper, massage his penis through the fabric. Keep kissing him, too. After you've opened his fly, slip your hand in

around his penis and testicles to protect them as you slide his pants down and off. Fondle him through his underpants before you lift the elastic over his stiff erection and glide them slowly down his thighs. You've just unwrapped a very special package.

78. Your nudity can be enhanced by leaving on one piece of jewelry or clothing; it tends to focus the erotic imagination. Try wearing only a long silk scarf to flutter against your breasts and his skin. Or leave on your stockings (roll them at the top so they stay up); you'll form a silky gate to paradise between your legs. Wear a pendant that hangs in your cleavage, or a single strand of pearls, and let it dangle against his chest or wrap it around his penis.

Above-the-elbow gloves are deliciously eccentric; or try wearing short gloves with the fingertips cut out so your stroking will produce two different sexy sensations. Don your lacy camisole or leave on your unbuttoned shirt. Wear only a slim gold chain around your waist or let your bracelets jangle disarmingly against his bare skin.

79. For contrast, don't take off anything at all — except your panties — and let him struggle with your clothes to "ravage" you. A very sexy man introduced me to this wonderful game by "ravaging" me one hot

Saturday afternoon without removing any of my clothes. I still don't understand how his engorged organ got past my panties, but it's amazing how inventive a highly aroused man and his penis can be!

playful props

80. *Long hair.* Wind it around his penis gently, then let it loosen by itself. Allow your hair to brush back and forth across his genitals.

81. *Washable body paint.* Re-create that wonderful scene from *Cousin, Cousine* by painting lovely designs all over his body and yours. After some Technicolor lovemaking, wash each other off in the bath.

82. *Erotic oils.* Let him watch you massage some onto your vaginal lips. Then invite him to slide his penis against you. Rub a tingly oil all over his genitals, especially into the slit at the top of the glans.

83. *Silk scarf.* Touch him only with the scarf. Use it as a hand covering while you stroke him. Rub it back

and forth between his thighs. Wrap it around his penis or testicles. Use it to tie his hands or feet together.

84. *Mirrors.* If you don't have one mounted next to or over your bed, make love while standing in front of whatever mirror is available. Press yourself against it occasionally to enjoy the cool, smooth sensation on your skin.

85. *Feathers.* Have a wide assortment at the ready: a feather duster, a boa, a quill, a peacock feather. Brush and tickle him unmercifully. Especially vulnerable to the feather touch are the face, neck, nipples, navel, inner thighs, backs of the knees, and of course the penis, scrotum, and rear end.

86. *Fruit.* A cherry or several berries inserted in your vagina make a delightful invitation to an adventurous snack. Push a peeled banana inside you and invite him to eat it out. Or mash the banana first (or peaches or papaya), stuff the puree inside your vagina, and let him smoosh his penis around in it.

87. *Spreadables.* Follow the lead of the ancient Roman courtesans and spread honey on your nipples, vag-

inal lips, and clitoris and let him lick it off. Whipped cream is another luscious enticement. Don't forget to spread some honey or cream on him, too; he'll make a lovely "candied apple" or "ice cream cone."

88. *Ice.* Put some small ice cubes in your mouth and suck his penis.

89. *Popsicle.* Get his favorite flavor Popsicle (or Froz-Fruit bar), give it a few preliminary sucks and licks for erotic effect, and then let him watch you masturbate with it. When either you or he can't stand the tension anymore, remove the Popsicle and invite him to fuck your shockingly icy vagina. A treat he'll never forget.

waterplay

Water is the most sensuous of all the natural elements; it almost oozes sex. Use it as a catalyst to create a whole new world of sensual delights.

90. After he's showered, dry him off with your tongue.

$91.$ *Bath #1.* After a hard day's work, invite him into a hot bubble bath. Use several scented candles instead of the harsh bathroom lights, put on some dreamy music, and sip a heady wine or champagne. Lather each other up — and down.

$92.$ *Bath #2.* For this one, you are the bather and he is the bathee. Get him wet but turn the water off while you soap him all over with sandalwood-, pine-, or mint-scented soap. Shower him off. Immediately run a very hot bath and let him soak in some masculine-flavored oil. Bring on the candles and the mood music and read erotic stories to him, or do a striptease, or masturbate for him while you murmur sexy promises about what's in store after his bath.

$93.$ *Bath #3.* Invite him to join you for a hot and sweaty workout. Follow it with an invigorating shower; lather him all over and give him a vigorous head massage when you wash his hair. Wrap him in a Turkish towel and lead him to the bed for a relaxing baby oil massage.

body parts

Just like you, he has lots of erogenous zones all over his body. If you explore thoroughly, you'll be sure to discover all of them and probably create some new ones!

94. *Eyelids.* A soft kiss, light lick, or gentle caress on your man's sensitive lids is a very intimate and unusual gesture. The exquisite closeness it creates will carry into the rest of your lovemaking and raise the level of intensity a few notches.

95. *Ears.* In many men, there is a direct connection between the ear and the penis. Plug into it and watch him sizzle. Suck, lick, nibble, and blow on the lobe and tender inner portions of the ear. For special effect, point your tongue and slide it in and out of the ear cavity; it feels marvelous and will make him think of sliding moistly in and out of you.

96. *Neck.* I have found that the crease under a man's chin and the skin over his esophagus and Adam's apple are especially sensitive areas and respond very nicely to sucking and licking. You might try alternating these activities with nibbling on the tendons extending

from ears to shoulders. When you've made him very hot, keep it up just a little longer; you'll make his penis tingle.

97. *Hair.* The right kind of hair-pulling can be very erotic. Grab him by the hair at the back of his head, draw his head back, and lick or love-bite his outstretched neck. Tell him how delicious he is.

98. *Armpits.* Any part of the body that is protected by hair or other body parts and is not usually exposed is exquisitely sensitive. Obviously the armpit qualifies as one of the premiere hot spots. Don't miss it. Stroking, licking, nuzzling, and nibbling produce delicious sensations and will usually have him writhing about in ecstasy, begging you to let him get inside you.

99. *Nipples.* Just like yours, a man's nipples are erotically sensitive. The difference is that, while the sensations he arouses in your nipples flow to and inflame other parts of your body and you love to have your rosy buds stimulated for long periods, a man's reaction to nipple massage is more localized, sharper, and wears thin much faster. Do unto his nipples as you would have him do unto yours, and you're off to a great start; but don't keep it up so long that it starts to feel more like irritation than lovely stimulation.

Suck, lick, and nibble. Pull the nipple out with your lips or teeth (gently!) and let it go. Circle it with your tongue, flick your tongue back and forth over it. Blow on it. Roll his nipples between your fingers. Squeeze them. Pull on them. Slather them with whipped cream or honey and lick it off. Add a few gentle strokes to his penis now and then to help diffuse the powerful sensations. Then move on to something else while he's still begging for more.

100. *Navel.* Here's another juicy spot to stick your tongue in. Massage, lick, and suck the surrounding area first, saving the slippery insertion for last. Tease him by tickling the surrounding hairs with your fingers and breath. Then thrust your pointed tongue in and out of his navel. Or pour in a little wine or honey and suck/lick it out.

101. *Spine.* I'll bet you never thought of the backbone as an erogenous zone. But men have sensitive nerves along the spine, especially at the tailbone, that seem to be directly connected to the genitals. Send erotic messages to his penis by traveling down his spine with your mouth and tongue. Bite gently, lick insistently, suck hungrily. Pay special attention to the very end of his spine, the tailbone, and stick your tongue in the crease of his buttocks while you're there.

$102.$ *Inner thighs.* That soft, protected area on the inside of his thighs, from above the knee to the crotch, is a hotbed of sexy sensations. And of course the higher up you go, the hotter he gets. Caress lightly, press firmly, tickle gently. Lap your tongue over the sensitive skin. Suck and nibble on the underlying tendon, especially right where it connects at the crotch. The spot where inner thigh meets pelvis is the most responsive to erotic stimulation. So spend some quality time there, and farther up the pelvic bone as well, before arriving at his now-quivering penis.

$103.$ *Hands.* The hands and fingers are made to be especially sensitive and discriminating of different textures and sensations. Use your fingernails to inscribe small circles on the palms of your man's hands. Hold his hand in yours and lick the palm while staring into his eyes. Suck each finger as though it were a small penis. Tease his fingertips with gentle scrapings of your teeth. Lick the backs of his hands, too, and circle his wrists with your tongue. Thrust your tongue in and out between his fingers and their base, and suck on his knuckles.

When his hand is nicely sensitized, you may want to guide it to your breast and move it in slow circles around your nipples, or pull it lower to trace his palm lightly across your pubic hair. He'll probably take over from there.

1 04. *Feet.* You *know* how sensitive and ticklish feet are. Use your mouth, tongue, and fingernails here as you did on his hands, paying special attention to the toes. Slide your tongue between them and suck, nibble, and pull on them as you would his penis. Some men will even ejaculate from a good toe sucking. But don't forget the soles, as they are extremely sensitive. Ancient acupuncturists felt that the upper part of the heel, just below the Achilles tendon, was the area affecting sexual response. Try massaging this area with your fingertips or applying pressure with your lips, tongue, and teeth. He'll have a new erogenous zone—created by you.

1 05. *Buttocks.* The adorable rear that looks so good in tight jeans fairly begs to be cupped in your sensuous hands. Don't miss the opportunity to give both of you a super-sexy treat. Start with a bun massage; then pull the skin tight and scrape your nails over his taut cheeks. Tickle the baby-fine hairs at his tailbone and massage the base of his spine. Pinch and bite his buns. Kiss, suck, and lick them. If you really want to drive him wild, reach around to stroke his penis at the same time. There's something so primitive,

yet so comforting, about a sensuous massage and kiss to the rear; neither of you may want to move on to anything else!

106. *Anus.* The anus is one of the most sensitive spots on his body. And you shouldn't leave it out of your erotic playtime just because you have misgivings about its other functions. When you start viewing it as just another part of the body (a very sensitive one at that), you'll begin to see the incredibly erotic possibilities latent there.

Feces come into the anal area only when you're just about to have a bowel movement. Just make sure you're both freshly bathed, and you'll have nothing to worry about. Honestly. And his reaction to your ministrations will make it well worth overcoming any inhibitions you might have.

A gentle fingertip massage to the surface of the anus is lovely, especially if you continue it down a little farther toward his scrotum, too. Pinch or blow on it, and yes, even lick it. The moisture you produce there will make it easier to insert the tip of your pinky into his anus and massage inside with circular motions and an easy in-and-out thrusting. An even sexier way of accomplishing this is to wet your finger in your own vaginal juice before inserting it in his rear. (*But don't put it back in your vagina after it's been in his anus.*) Again, you can put the icing on the cake by massaging his penis simultaneously.

To be really safe, you should try anal pleasures only with someone whose sexual and general health you are sure of.

107. *Scrotum and testicles.* The scrotum, which is the pouch of skin holding the testicles, is extremely sensitive, so use the lightest of touches here. Stroke softly, lick, or blow light breaths over the skin. Some men like it when you take one or both of their testicles in your mouth and suck gently. Or lightly massage them with one hand while stroking his penis with the other.

Many men love to have you pull on their testicles while you're massaging their penis. Either encircle the top of the scrotum, right up next to his body, with your thumb and forefinger, or pinch both sides of the scrotum together between the testicles, and pull down. Don't jerk. Pull easily and gently, in rhythm with the strokes you're giving his penis. You should know that pulling his testicles down firmly is one way to forestall ejaculation; this trick may come in handy for those times when you're not quite ready for the show to end.

108. *Perineum.* The small area between the anus and the scrotum is one of the most secret, sexy spots on a man. (You have one of these spots too, between your anus and vulva.) Even the simple pressure of your finger there will send waves of pleasure throughout his genital area. While you're massaging his penis or anus, use your finger to exert firm pressure on the perineum and move it in a circular or back-and-forth pattern. Your man probably doesn't even know he has this delicious little spot (it's similar to your G spot). He'll be grateful to you for "pointing it out" to him!

using other parts of your body

The hands, mouth, and tongue are the usual appendages applied to a man's skin. Why not try something different occasionally? Use every part of your body as a tool for pleasure. Be imaginative. Be daring. Be provocative.

109. *Eyelashes.* Bat your lashes against his cheeks, ears, lips, underarms, nipples, tummy, penis, behind his knees, on the bottoms of his feet. Alternate between fast and slow flicks.

110. *Hair.* If you have long hair, wrap it around

his penis. Then release and let it unravel slowly as you pull away. Dangle it loosely all over his body.

| | | . *Teeth.* Bite him gently anywhere you would kiss him. Take hold of him by the hair, bend his head to you, and bite his lower lip. Bite and suck on his neck like a *vamp*ire. Chew on the inside of his elbows and knees. Love-bite his nipples, belly button, and scrumptious buns. Bite his ears and toes, alternating with torrid tongue thrusts. Eat him up all over!

| | 2 . *Nipples.* Your nipples can be used to give as well as receive pleasure. Trail your erect nipples over your man's entire body, taking the time to stop occasionally for a wiggle and jiggle over sensitive spots. Guide one or both nipples into all his cavities and crevices—ears, mouth, hollow of the neck, underarms, navel, crease between thigh and genitals, spaces between the toes, backs of his knees, crease at the bottom of his buns, anus, crack between his "cheeks," hollow of lower back. Press your nipples against his and roll them together with your fingers. Caress his lips with your nipples and let him lick them for a while. Wind up this lovely treat with several seductive passes over and around his genitals. The sight as well as the sensation will drive him wild.

1 1 3. *Pubic hair.* A delightful way to tickle your man and arouse his animal passion is to trail your pubic hair and pelvis over his whole body. Start by having him lie on his stomach and climb astride his shoulders. Slide, rotate, or bump and grind your way down his backside slowly and deliberately. You'll soon be wet and juicy, which will turn him on even more. When you reach his heel, put it between your vaginal lips and pump up and down as though it were a big penis. Insert each of his toes in your juicy vagina, too. When you turn him over and start progressing upward, you can handle his knee in the same way. Leave his penis for last as you make your erotic trip up over his stomach, chest, neck, chin, and nose.

If you want, you can give him a chance to relieve some of his sexual tension by situating your vulva over his mouth and letting him kiss and lick you for a while. Then insinuate yourself back down to his pelvis and rub up and down the shaft lightly with just your pubic hairs at first, slowly increasing the pressure till your whole wet vagina is giving him the thrill of his life and he's screaming "Fuck me, fuck me!" It's up to you whether you put him out of his "misery" right then or later.

1 1 4. *Feet.* Make sure they're clean first. A good pedicure doesn't hurt, either. Then use your feet to give him an all-over massage, just as though they were your hands. Besides being generally exotic, there are two very special attractions to this trick. (1) As you maneuver yourself and your feet around to the most comfortable and useful positions for massage, he gets some spectacular views of your vagina, from many erotic angles. (2) You can masturbate him with your feet and toes. Come as close as you can to putting the soles of your feet together, put his penis between them and rub up and down. Or hold his cock at its base with your big and second toe while sliding up and down the entire shaft and tweaking the tip with the same toes of your other foot. You can always use your own natural lubrication to make this even smoother and sexier.

115. *The sensuous massage.* There's nothing quite as inviting, languorous, and sensual as a slinky, full-body massage. Make sure the room is warm and you are both fresh and clean before situating your man on the bed or on a thick carpet. Both of you should be naked. Always use oil so your hands will slide smoothly and uninterruptedly over his tender skin. You can use massage oil or any vegetable oil scented with your favorite perfume or aromatherapy essence. Keep it warm over a candle throughout the entire massage.

As much as possible, use your entire hand — the palm

and the pressed-together fingers — to make contact with *all* the areas of your lover's body. You can start anywhere and use any kind of stroke as long as your movements are slow, steady, smooth, and in constant rhythm. Knead with your fingers, press with your palms, circle with your whole hand, pound gently with the sides of your hands, and slide your hands gently back to their starting position at the end of each stroke. Repeat each movement at least three times before moving on to a different stroke. Don't forget to spend a good deal of time on his head, hands, and feet; massage in these areas can elicit some of the most directly sexual responses from your mate.

To lend erotic accompaniment to the feel of your warmly insistent hands, add your hot breath or your cool, silky tongue to the stimulation of his neck, nipples, abdomen, inside of his arm or leg, or anywhere else you can think of. Keep up your slow, steady and sensuous movements for at least thirty minutes, and then, depending on both your moods, either towel him off and luxuriate in the quiet intimacy of the moment, or oil yourself down, too, slither up against him, and see what comes up.

what to do with his penis

116. *Holding it right.* Not having a penis puts us women at a big disadvantage when it comes to knowing how to make one feel good. But one of the biggest mistakes you can make is to assume that what feels wonderful on your clitoris and in your vagina will feel equally wonderful to his genitals. Wrong! In case you hadn't noticed, his penis is a completely different animal altogether. Whereas the general rule for most clitorises is "the gentler the better," for most penises it's "the firmer the better." So you should develop a grip for him something like the one you use on your tennis racket.

The most sensitive areas of the penis are the head, the rim around the bottom of the head, the long ridge running the length of the underside, and—probably the most sensitive spot—the slender string of skin connecting head to shaft on the underside. If you keep these hot spots in mind and use your fingers accordingly, you should have a very happy penis in your hands.

Some of the better ways to hold this lovely piece of equipment, depending on the direction from which you approach it, are: (1) Rest your index finger on the little thread of skin going from head to shaft; other fingers can line up along the underside ridge. Let your thumb lie against the rim of the shaft on the top side. (2) Place your thumb on the bottom of the underside ridge, while the rest of your fingers curl around the shaft, with your pinky resting against the rim of the shaft. (3) Make a ring with your thumb and index finger and slip it snugly around the base of the rim as a starting point.

117. *Stroking it right.* Now that your hand is strategically placed, it's time to get a little action going. Just three things to remember for the perfect stroke: do it firmly, do it smoothly, and do it in a steady rhythm.

If you want him to climax this way, increase your speed as he nears orgasm. But when he actually get there, stop moving your hand. Either grasp him more tightly and just hold on, or relax your grip completely and let your hand act as a cradle.

If you have other plans for his penis while it's still hard, simply remove your hand gently and smoothly when you feel him getting too excited. Be sure to distract his attention right away with a deep kiss or a deep plunge into your wet vagina.

variations on the basic stroke

118. Knead his penis between both your hands as though it were a piece of dough.

119. Roll it between your palms.

120. Stroke the underside with your palm as you press his penis against his pelvis.

121. Make two rings with the thumb and index finger of each hand. Place them next to each other in the middle of his shaft. Gently pull outward in both directions at once.

122. Make two rings as above. But this time put them both at the base of his penis. Slide your top hand up toward the glans, letting it come off the end completely. Then replace it at the base and repeat the stroke. The "ring" of your other hand should exert pressure downward as the top hand moves upward. Keep repeating these strokes till he begs for mercy.

123. Roll or thump his penis against your belly, thigh, or face.

124. Press your breasts together and let him slide his well-oiled penis between them. Occasionally, he can rub it across your nipples. Or he can alternate his thrusting with sucking on your nipples. Or while he's busy sliding between your breasts, you can stimulate your nipples yourself. He'll enjoy watching this. Or at the end of each stroke, let his penis emerge from between your breasts and into your waiting mouth.

125. If your man has a high level of appreciation for women's bottoms, he'll no doubt enjoy rubbing his penis between the cheeks of your behind. Lubricate yourself there and present your derriere from a kneeling position or by lying on your stomach with pillows beneath your hips.

126. Here's one you may like even better than he does. Lie on your back and prop up your pelvis very high with pillows. Invite him to kneel between your legs and move his penis slowly over and between your vaginal lips. No penetration allowed!

127. Lie on your back with pillows beneath your pelvis, and press your thighs tightly together. He should then straddle your legs with his and let his penis hang straight down between your lubricated thighs. He can thrust up and down in this silken vise for a while and then move in closer so that he rubs against your clitoris and vaginal lips as he goes up and down. A more relaxed position for this juicy little game is one where you lie on your sides, either facing each other or with your back toward him. If you use the position where he comes through from the rear, you can fondle his penis each time it appears in front of you.

128. For an extra little treat, press on his "G spot" while you're caressing his penis. The area between his anus and scrotum is called the perineum. When you press there, you are stimulating his prostate; for him, this feels similar to the way G-spot stimulation feels for you. Use your forefinger and press firmly and in rhythm while you stroke his penis with your other hand. If it's comfortable, you can curl the other fingers of your pressing hand around the base of his organ, using them to keep the penile skin taught. This sort of handiwork usually makes for a more deeply felt and longer-lasting orgasm.

129. Another thing you can do while rubbing his penis is to fondle his testicles. Cup them gently in your hand as you caress the base of his penis with your fingertips. Or, with thumb and forefinger on either side, press your fingers together between his testicles and pull down gently in rhythm with your stroking. Or use the ring technique around the base of his scrotum and again pull down rhythmically. Whichever technique you choose, use firm pressure but *don't squeeze too hard.*

130. Remember the delightful nipple-stroking you gave him? (See #112.) Ask him to do the same to you with his penis. All that stimulation will drive you *both* wild.

131. Surprise him by reaching into his pants and fondling him while he's reading, talking on the phone, watching TV, cooking, or washing the dishes.

132. Every man's fantasy is to have an incredibly sensuous dream about a beautiful, lusty lady making love to him and then wake up to find it's actually happening. So sometime in the middle of the night, while he's sleeping soundly, gently and slowly caress his penis; stroke it, squeeze it, roll it between your hands. Try to arouse his delicate organ without waking him. When he's nice and hard, slide him inside you and make drowsily sweet love to him.

133. The first time you see your man again after a period of separation (even if it's only been since this morning when you both left for work), greet him with some bold and sensuous eye/hand coordination. First lock eyes with him, sometimes best accomplished by whispering, "Look at me, darling." Then slither over to him, never taking your eyes from his. Let your eyes tell him you have sex on your mind.

When you reach him, gently take hold of his penis and start massaging. Be sure to keep your eyes on his the whole time — fix him with your burning gaze. Continue stroking and eventually free his now-hard member from his pants so he can feel skin-to-skin contact. Still keep your eyes locked with his.

It'll be up to you whether to finish this by kneeling down to take him in your mouth, or slipping him into your panty-less vagina while standing there, or backing away and pulling him with your sultry eyes into the bedroom.

134. Here's a nice combination. Start by stroking his penis into a state of throbbing arousal. Then stop and truss him up, spreadeagled on the bed. Don't touch him anymore, but instead fondle your own breasts and vagina as sensuously as you possibly can. Let him watch you writhe, shiver, and moan, finally exploding in a shattering orgasm while he lies there helpless. This sexy sight will drive him absolutely wild. Untie him and have wild, passionate sex.

135. Here's a variation on a technique I learned from a wonderful book called *ESO: How You and Your Lover Can Give Each Other Hours of Extended Orgasm.* After your man has been tied for a while and has reached fever pitch, sit astride his chest with your back to his face. Firmly grasp the root of his penis with one hand and, with the other, stroke upward very rapidly and sharply. Wait for the space of one heartbeat and repeat. Give him about ten of these and then ten more of the same stroke but all in rapid succession, no pausing in between. Alternate these two stroking groups (one with pauses, one without) for five to eight minutes or until he screams for mercy. Finally, give him a spectacular orgasm by way of your hand, mouth, or vagina. Be sure to untie him quickly after his orgasm so his whole body doesn't get stiff and sore. Let him lie there and bask in the glory of you.

136. If you are bringing your man to climax by

hand, you can simply loosen your pressure and stop pumping while he's actually in the throes of orgasm (as recommended earlier), or you can try another method that may extend his orgasm briefly; this depends on the individual fella. Try it and see how your man reacts. Keep up your stroking as he reaches orgasm, but lightly. After he's ejaculated, confine your efforts to his scrotum and "G spot." Lightly pull on the shaft of his penis (stay away from the head) and massage his scrotum and perineum. This should feel to him as though you're "milking" him for even more juice and more contractions.

137. There are many delightful ways to arouse your man's penis without touching it, and often this is the most powerful stimulant of all. Suck each of his fingers or toes slowly and provocatively. Thrust your tongue in and out of his ear. Lick his nipples and lift your head as you suck them upward and outward. Let your tongue dart in and out of the crack of his behind; slither it around his anus and underneath to his testicles. Use your fingernails to excite any leftover spots!

"The moment came when

I wanted you physically.

Without warning I put

my tongue out and

slithered it along the

gossamer smooth stem that

was slightly curved, the

skin taut. I was trembling

too now and I found it

hard to breathe."

—Compiled by Maren Sell,

The Pleasure of Loving

4

oral
treats

for a man, there is absolutely nothing to equal the ecstasy of a woman lovingly sucking and licking his penis. To him, it is the most intimate, loving, ego-gratifying, and supremely sexy gesture a woman can perform. No other sexual act allows him to fantasize in quite the same way; he can imagine that the woman with her mouth around him is completely dominated by his awe-inspiring masculinity, that she is his to command, that she loves him totally and without reserve, that she is his sexual slave. This line of thinking turns him on tremendously and should result in some great reciprocal tongue work on you or the hottest sex you've ever had. So keep in mind that great mouth work produces honey for both bears.

Many women feel squeamish about putting their mouths and tongues on a man's genitals. Others are afraid of it because they don't know what to do. But genital kisses are some of the most wonderful things about sexual intimacy. And most women find that, after their first few successful tries, they develop a real taste for this lusty occupation.

The one thing to be careful about is sharing oral sex with someone you don't know well. Though many researchers believe this to be a low risk for transmitting HIV, it's always better to be safe by avoiding oral/genital contact with untried lovers — especially contact with semen. But if you and your man are *sure* of each other's health, then absolutely add the wonders of genital kissing to your sexual repertoire.

There are three things to remember when putting lips to penis. I call them the three C's.

1. *Crave it.*
2. *Concentrate.*
3. *Continuous movement.*

craving it

When speaking of the best oral sex they've ever had, men invariably mention that it was the woman's passion about what she was doing that made it so outstanding. "I could tell she really loved licking my penis, and it made me feel special." "She was even more excited than I was. I had to beg her to stop." "She made me feel like my penis was the tastiest lollipop she'd ever had in her mouth, and she was savoring every lick."

Once again, attitude is everything. You must *really want* to pleasure him this way; you must *know* that you can. Develop a passion for that extraordinary and mysterious piece of equipment that dangles between his legs. Show him with your excitement that you crave the feel of his penis in your mouth. Relish it. Treat it like a beautiful and sacred tool of pleasure. Delight in his masculinity, and he will delight in your femininity.

concentrating
Focus on your task. Don't let your attention or your passion wander. This keeps the intensity high.

continuous movement
Do everything continuously, smoothly, and evenly. No sudden jerking or abrupt shifts. Keep the action and the juices flowing.

1 38. Really hot oral sex takes caring and preparation. Look at his gorgeous, hard erection and savor the thought that now you're actually going to get to taste, kiss, and suck it, like an ice cream cone! And he's gonna love it.

Stroke his penis lovingly with your hands and let him anticipate the coming attraction. Remember the brain is the hottest erogenous zone. Tell him how sexy his penis is and how hot it makes you. Tell him just what you're going to do to it.

Start by licking the head of his penis. Find the ridge that runs down the underside and run your tongue along it and across it. Point your tongue and flick it over the ridge between the head and the shaft. (This is usually his most sensitive spot.) While this is going on, you should stroke the rest of his penis, his thighs, stomach—anywhere—with your free hand.

Visualize your mouth as a very imaginative and agile vagina. Then open your mouth, cover your teeth with your lips (so you won't hurt him), and slide his penis slowly inside. Let it rest on your tongue. Now move your head up and down smoothly and *continuously*. (Don't blow his enjoyment and your concentration by stopping and starting!) Remember to keep your teeth covered and increase your speed gradually.

Put your hand around the base of his penis and move it up and down in rhythm with the movement of your mouth. They should both go up and down together. While he's in your mouth, you can also wiggle your tongue back and forth across his quivering shaft and probe into the slit on the top. Delicious!

139. Another great tongue trick is to move it in circles around and around his penis while it slides merrily up and down. Not easy but worth it. Occasionally, you can just suck on him like a piece of hard candy. Use your other hand to caress his inner thighs, scrotum, anus, tummy, or whatever you can reach.

140. Gently lick his testicles and take them one at a time into your mouth. Move your tongue languidly around each one. This is very erotic for him and very few women (if any) will have delighted him this way.

141. Another tremendous turn-on for him, if he's not too shy or ticklish to let you do it, is to lick the crack of his behind while you massage his penis. (For health reasons, it's probably best to steer clear of the anal opening itself.)

142. That small area between his scrotum and anus, the perineum, is very sensitive to tongue work, too. It's so sensitive, in fact, that you may want to start with a few very gentle licks and hold his thighs down (or up) to protect yourself from his rapturous writhing.

143. While giving the basic genital kiss, insert one wet finger into his anus, very gently. Move it around in circles and in and out.

144. Lightly massage his perineum while sucking his penis. But watch out that this doesn't make him come sooner than you want him to!

145. Hold his penis in your mouth by sucking

firmly and shake your head at the same time. This gives him a nice little tingle.

146. Men love it when you alternate your mouth with your vagina. So, during your expert rendition of mouth music, give his penis an occasional, one-stroke dip into the deep well of your desire.

147. Although you always want to protect his delicate organ from your possibly too fervent fangs, there are times when your teeth make a nice prop. Hold his penis in your mouth sideways, like an ear of corn, and slide your teeth and tongue up and down the shaft. You can even give it a gentle nip now and then, but be sure to keep it *light!*

148. For an extra added taste treat, eat a banana, peach, berries, orange, or other juicy fruit while eating him. Rub the juice all over his penis and lick it off, or simply keep the food in your mouth while you give him a fruity genital kiss.

149. Dip his penis into a jar of honey, jam, maple syrup, cream, or melted chocolate (cooled off a little) and lap it up. Yum!

150. Try using a strong mint-flavored mouth-wash just before you get into bed. Your tangy tongue and mouth on his delicate penile skin will cause quite a sensation.

151. Surprise him now and again. While you're both innocently watching TV (all your clothes on, of course!), unzip him and suck away to your heart's content.

152. Sneak up on your man while he's on the phone to Mom or the boss or the landlord. Let your mouth make him hard as iron.

153. In the middle of the night, wake him up with your tantalizing tongue.

154. One delicious man I know tells me that receiving oral sex while standing or kneeling is one of the most ecstatic sensations a man can experience. His upright position apparently intensifies the exquisite pressure in his penis; and the sight of a lusty woman kneeling before him, "worshiping" his organ, puts the frosting on the cake. Play around with the best positions for this to accommodate your respective heights; he kneels on the edge of the bed and you kneel on the floor, or he stands on the bed or a chair and you stand on the floor, or he kneels on the floor and you sit on the floor with your legs wrapped around his knees. (What a view for him!) Caress his legs, inner thighs, buttocks, and stomach as you suck him passionately. Rub your nipples against his legs. Stop occasionally to tell him how gorgeous his erection is and how hot it's making you.

155. Hum while you have his penis in your mouth. The vibrations feel divine.

156. Of course, every man's fantasy is to have a beautiful woman give him genital kisses under the dining table. If you can pull this off in a dark restaurant, good for you. But it will work almost as well in the privacy of your own dining room. Make sure the table is dressed in a floor-length cloth to provide just the right touch of secrecy and forbidden "fruit."

157. The *Kama Sutra*, the classic Indian text on lovemaking, details the art of oral sex at great length. Here is one particular sequence of events that I have found especially exciting. First, take your man's penis

in your mouth sideways and move it gently between your lips. Then hold it with your fingers while pressing its sides with your lips and teeth slightly. Kiss it as if drawing it out. Push his lovely member a little farther into your mouth, still pressing with your lips, and slowly pull it out again. Suck it as you would his lower lip. Then lick it all over, giving special attention to its head. Next, take his penis halfway into your mouth and forcefully kiss and suck it. Finally, draw it in as far as it will go, press the end against the roof of your mouth, and suck as though you would swallow it. He'll be swallowed up in ecstasy.

158. *The famous and fabulous "69."* Licking your man's penis while letting him kiss your lovely vagina is one of the greatest treats you can offer him. Men are completely fascinated with the delicious naughtiness and utter hedonism of this tasty maneuver. There are as many variations to 69 as there are to intercourse positions and kisses. Try them all; he'll adore you for it.

A particularly nice refinement on 69 is to use your mouth as you would your vagina. Imitate its contractions and sucking movements. Invite him to slide his tongue inside you and embrace it with your PC muscle at the same time that you are sucking on his penis. Let your mouth and vagina contract and relax simultaneously in waves. Establish an easy rhythm and keep it up until he begs for mercy.

159. *Deep-throating.* Linda Lovelace's famous technique is not as difficult as it looks, although it takes some practice. The key is to get your mouth and throat into proper position (a long, straight line) by lying on your back with your head hanging off the edge of the bed. Take a deep breath first because your man's penis is going to temporarily block your breathing. Don't worry, you can breathe on each out-stroke. And don't be con cerned about gagging. If you feel the urge to gag, just swallow. With practice you'll find that the gagging feeling will go away, and your man will be coming back for more.

 160. *Swallowing semen.* This can be one of the most intimate, satisfying, and erotic things you'll ever do for your lover. Almost every man derives intense fulfillment from having a sexy woman swallow his "sacred essence" with obvious pleasure. Just think how you'd feel if he lustily lapped up your juices and swallowed them with delight!

Semen is composed mainly of protein and sugar; it's completely natural and utterly harmless (as long as you know he's healthy). So every love goddess who's worth her salt should learn and practice this fine art. The secret is to think of his juice as a tasty, intimate gift and to swallow it all in one gulp; that way it bypasses most of your taste buds. Most important, look and act as if you loved it! Otherwise the whole effect is ruined and he'll feel uncomfortably self-conscious.

If you just can't get into the idea of swallowing semen, there are ways to avoid it while still giving him the pleasure of having an orgasm while in your mouth. Without making a big deal of it, just hold the semen in your mouth and make an *elegant* exit to the bathroom to spit it out. Or have a washcloth or tissue handy, turn away for a moment, and *unobtrusively* empty his juices into it.

Since few women can, or want to, swallow their lover's semen, and since most men value the act so highly, here's your opportunity to create a lasting impression and form a very special bond with your man.

161. Another terribly loving and sexy thing to do is to gently lap at his penis *after* he's had his orgasm. This works especially well as an exquisite contrast following very lusty or animalistic sex. It's the whipped cream on the cake's frosting.

"For what is the beloved? She is that which I myself am not. In the act of love, I am pure male, and she is pure female. She is she, and I am I, and clasped together with her, I know how perfectly she is not me, how perfectly I am not her, how utterly we are two, the light and the darkness, and how infinitely and eternally not-to-be-comprehended by either of us is the surpassing One we make."
—D. H. Lawrence

5
the
main
course

the sublimely simple act of penis thrusting into vagina is the most primitive, the most all-encompassing, and the most magical of all the types of sexual interplay—an ecstasy like no other, a divinely wordless communication, the supreme act of trust and love. Yet many of us allow this wonderful mystery to become a repetitious bore. Many men simply pump up and down till they have an orgasm and then roll over for a snore. Many women just lie motionless till he's finished and then wonder why they feel unfulfilled. Some of us are inventive and ardent lovers in every other way but fail to bring the same excitement to the act of copulation.

Great fucking is an art. It takes practice, imagination, and passion. It requires concentration and control as well as the ability to let go completely. It needs a lot of knowing and a little intuition. It needs, obviously, a man and a woman. But never make the mistake of just lying back and expecting your man to do all the work. It's not just the man's show. To make intercourse truly sensational, you must take at least an equal part in the action.

So do something extra to make it exciting and electric. When he least expects it, apply a little imagination and really drive him—and yourself—wild! Here are some basics to remember.

Sexual intercourse is an intimate act of *union.* Through joining your bodies, the two of you become truly one. As a woman, you are the one most likely to recognize and understand this magical feeling of oneness. So if you can communicate this to your lover, you'll have raised his enjoyment—and yours—to a new level. Don't try to use words. Unless he's unusually sensitive, he won't hear you at this very physical point. Try to slow him down so you can communicate physically. Let the feeling shine from your eyes as you stare deeply into his; let your moans and sighs be deep and expressive of completion; let the movements of your hips welcome and cherish the union of your bodies. Eventually, he'll get the picture.

The most vivid sensations are a result of *deep penetration* and *intense friction.* Enjoy as many positions as you want, but during each session, make sure you maneuver into at least one that provides for a very snug fit and some super-deep thrusts.

Now is the time to make use of those *agile vaginal muscles* you've been exercising. Hold him deep inside you with the grasp of your muscles. Push him out provocatively. Contract and release rapidly, then slowly and sensually. Let those talented inner muscles ripple over his penis tantalizingly. Both the incredible physical sensations and the thought that your hot, lovely vagina is undulating like crazy—for him—will drive any man to the heights of passion.

Never fake an orgasm. Why? Because he'll probably be able to tell. Because you're only cheating yourself. Because if you don't show him how to satisfy you properly, he'll just keep on being ineffectual for you, and the problem will get worse.

Don't destroy his ego with accusations. Just say something like, "Honey, I didn't quite make it yet. Would you please rub my clitoris?" Or simply masturbate yourself while still kissing and stroking him. Later on, when things have quieted down, you can calmly discuss what needs to be changed or improved. At these times, always make sure to reinforce his virility through your words and actions, and be gentle, loving, and *informative.* He'll just be frustrated further if you don't let him know how to give you an orgasm. And so will you.

Movement is everything. It goes without saying that, while he's pumping into you, your hips should be thrusting up to meet his. Believe me, there's nothing sexier than an undulating pelvis. But while all this bumping and grinding is going on, make sure to keep kissing, licking, biting, stroking, and caressing the rest of his body. Show your man that you're so hot for him you can't keep your hands or mouth off any part of him. Let him know he's gotten you so excited you can't control yourself; your hands and mouth are everywhere, your hips are pounding wildly, and your moans and sighs speak of the deepest ecstasy. He has set you on fire and you want to utterly consume his unbearably sexy body and soul. Get the picture?

And finally, don't forget that condom!

All of the many possible positions for intercourse are really just variations on the basic five: the missionary (man on top), the woman on top, rear entry, side by side, and sitting face-to-face.

missionary position

Although unfortunately named, this is one of the most comfortable positions, especially for prolonged intercourse. It affords a great deal of control and allows you to mouth-kiss, embrace, and watch the excitement on your lover's face while you let him see the burning passion on yours. The only disadvantages are that his arms may get tired, your freedom of movement is somewhat restricted, and penetration is not as deep as in some other positions. But the benefits make up for it.

162. Give him a warm and inviting welcome by guiding him inside you with your hands, gently and caressingly. If he is uncircumcised, this also gives you a chance to peel back the foreskin so he'll have maximum exposure.

163. Don't just lie there, do something! Thrust your hips up to meet his with every stroke. Imagine your quivering vagina is devouring his throbbing organ. Different angles will give shallower or deeper penetration and will make your clitoris meet his pubic bone in all sorts of delicious ways. Rotating your hips in a circular motion will also supply lovely sensations for both of you. So gyrate those hips, you hussy!

164. For even deeper penetration, open your legs wide and lift them up. The higher you can go, the deeper he can thrust. Then embrace him with your legs and push him into you with each stroke. If you are fairly agile, you can put your feet on his buttocks and push him in, creating an even more acute angle. In this position, you might feel his penis against your cervix or G spot. Go for it!

165. Now's the time to cash in on your PC muscle–tightening efforts. Milk him with your vagina by tightening and pushing out in rhythm with his strokes, or twitch even faster, or hold the contraction for a few strokes and then push out for a few more. This will drive him right up the wall.

166. To slow things down a bit—you want this

exquisite agony to go on for at least a few more hours, don't you? — completely relax your vaginal muscles and put your legs down flat alongside his or even underneath them. This will make for shallower thrusts. But keep your hips rocking so he'll know you're still very interested.

167. Another nice way to give him a rest while keeping him hot is to ask (or motion for) him to stop while *you* do all the thrusting. Make sure he's deep inside you first. Then bend your knees, keep your feet on the bed, and push yourself up enough to do some bumps and grinds on your own. Not only does he get to relax, but he can also concentrate fully on the delicious sensations you're giving him — with the added bonus of watching your lustily thrashing body!

168. A modification to #167 that you can continue when he starts moving again is what I call the "stripper's bump." Keep your knees bent, feet flat on the bed, but lower your hips to the mattress. Now press the small of your back into the bed while your pelvis thrusts upward, then relax. Repeat this motion slowly and hypnotically; he'll soon be mesmerized.

169. *Knee-chest position.* This variation on the basic missionary position is a dandy for both of you. Raise your legs so that your knees are pressed to your chest and drape your legs over his shoulders. He can penetrate much more deeply (your vagina actually gets longer), and you will benefit from the increased pressure and friction on your clitoris and vaginal lips.

170. One of my favorite positions is a combination of the knee-chest and the one in which both your legs lie flat down beside him. You simply put one of your knees to your chest and drape your leg over his shoulder, while the other leg lies flat, outside his torso. In this position, you are almost doing the splits, and you are very exposed as well as very coy. There's something psychologically thrilling, for both of you, about this sort of brassy vulnerability. He will feel like a lusty conquering hero, spreading open the legs of a sweet maiden; and you'll simply love being "taken."

171. One branch of yoga, called tantra, teaches that sexual union is a pathway to enlightenment. A tantric kissing technique, to be used during intercourse, involves the especially sweet saliva that is produced during lovemaking. Sometime during foreplay or at the beginning of intercourse, tell your man that you are going to make a special juice for him in your mouth. Tell him that it happens just before you

climax and that you will give it to him with your tongue so he can suck the sweetness of the orgasm he gives you. To do this, place the tip of your tongue against the roof of your mouth, just behind your front teeth, as your climax approaches. Then put your tongue in his mouth and let him suck your special nectar. He won't forget the image or the sensation of this erotic gift.

woman-on-top position

Knowing how to "ride" your man is one of the great secrets of expert lovemaking. For you, it's exciting to be in control for a change and to know you can do anything you want. You will also be very deeply penetrated.

You'll be giving your man quite a thrill too. Here's why. (1) You are showing him he's made you so mad with desire that you can't keep yourself from throwing caution and inhibition to the wind to "attack" him; a very exciting change for someone who always has to risk rejection and make the first or leading moves. (2) Best explained by one man I know: "When my woman gets on top of me, I can feast my eyes on her whole beautiful body. She's displaying it for me. I can watch her hips grind into me and her vagina devour my penis. I can see her beautiful breasts, nipples erect and glistening, sway and jiggle with every thrust. And I can reach up and play with them anytime I want. I run my hands down her smooth belly and over her pulsating clitoris. That's when I look up to see, best of all, the passion on her face." (3) His eager penis can reach very deeply into you. (4) He can rest while enjoying some truly exquisite sensations. (5) When you have your orgasm, he can feel the rippling of your vaginal muscles much more intensely than in any other position.

So every now and then, give your man an erotic treat—lusty you on top of lucky him!

172. *Woman-on-top foreplay.* Don't be in too much of a hurry to get him inside you. Take advantage of the opportunity to display your sexy body and get him really hot first. With him on his back and you on your knees, gracefully arc one leg over him and balance your weight on your knees and feet. Keep your back straight and breasts thrust out so he gets the full effect. Then lean forward to take some of your weight on your hands. Take his penis in hand and rub your moist vaginal lips and clitoris against it. Tease the head of his penis by sliding it back and forth across your opening, occasionally inserting just the tip and taking it out again. Finally, slide him in gently and slowly, with or without hands. Now that you're all set, there are several things you can do.

173. Lean forward. Rest on your hands or elbows; hands on the bed or on his shoulders or chest. This position allows you to thrust your hips freely, and please do. Up and down, around and around, side to side, moving your whole body or just your pelvis. To monitor your pace, be sensitive to his responses, slowing down when he gets too excited. Nibble on his neck, ears, face, and lips. If you can comfortably reach them, suck his nipples, too.

174. Sit up straight, affording the deepest penetration and the fullest body display. From this position, you can grind your pelvis around and around and back and forth. But you should concentrate more on twitching the inside of your vagina. Here again, your newly fit vaginal muscles should come into play, squeezing, pushing, and pulling, vibrating maddeningly.

175. When you feel especially sensuous, you can give him an extra treat by letting him see you play with your nipples and even masturbating yourself. This is a sight most men find highly erotic, and your increased gyrations will make him even hotter. Of course, you can invite him to do some of the stroking himself!

176. Ride him like you would a horse. Use your

best posting position and increase your speed with the excitement of the "race."

177. From this position, you can roll over into the missionary position without disconnecting; and it's nice to inject a little variety. But one of my favorite tricks is this. Stay on top and perform a 180-degree turn, so that you're facing his feet, then lean forward, bracing yourself with your hands between his legs, and start moving your body back and forth. It gets even better if you wrap one of your legs *underneath* his, giving him maximum penetration and a lovely view of your bouncing bottom (which he'll find hard not to fondle).

178. From the position described in #177, give him an extra treat by reaching down to massage his testicles; it's quite easy from here. You could also massage your clitoris at the same time, or rub his testicles against it, although you'll be getting a lot of stimulation of the whole vaginal area just from thrusting up against him. This position may sound a trifle strange and contorted, but don't knock it till you've tried it. Believe me, you'll both be getting the ride of your lives!

179. This one takes good balance and a little bit of practice but is well worth the effort. Squat over your man's thighs, placing your feet atop his thighs or pelvis, and inserting his penis deep inside you. Close your legs together. Then move your hips in circles over him, churning and undulating until you are both deeply satisfied.

rear entry

Yes, there are disadvantages to the rear entry positions; neither of you has a frontal view, and you can't hug and kiss. But the advantages are too exciting to miss. Your breasts are hanging free (they're more sensitive that way), and he can easily reach them. You get stimulation to the clitoris, vulva, the sensitive place between your vagina and anus, and your fanny. He gets extra stimulation on his scrotum, and both of you can enjoy the angle and depth of penetration. Besides, it's natural, lusty, and fun. If he's a fanny man or you have a particularly beautiful bottom, you should by all means "put on the dog" as a regular habit.

180. *The basic "doggy."* If you've seen dogs do it, you'll know just how to get into position for this one. Get on all fours and let your man come in from behind. He can be on his knees, too, or to make it even easier, he can stand on the floor *beside* the bed while you assume the doggy position in front of him on the bed. This per-

mits a lot of freedom of movement, and you can both get to rockin' and rollin' pretty well. Let your whole body move back and forth, and tip your hips so that your entire genital area makes contact with his pelvis and scrotum each time you "meet." You can also throw in a few hip swivels or reach one of your hands back to caress his flapping testicles.

He'll be unable to keep his hands off your delectable fanny, but encourage him to reach around to your clitoris and up to your swinging breasts, as well. When hanging down like this, your nipples are extra sensitive, and the increased fervor he'll produce in you by rubbing them will spur him on to even wilder thrusting.

181. You can also perform the "doggy" lying down. To facilitate the angle of entry and give you a little more room to undulate, put a pillow (or even two) under your hips. The higher your hips, the better the genital contact and the better the view for him. But be sure to keep your head far enough from the wall or headboard so his eager thrusts don't push you into it.

182. An interesting variation in the rear entry repertoire is the seated position. Ask your lover to sit on the edge of the bed or in a comfortable chair. You sit on top of him, facing away. He should put his hands up to steady you as you slowly descend onto his waiting penis. You can keep your legs inside his or spread them wide around his thighs. He won't be able to move much, so it's up to you to provide all the action. Hold on to his legs, the bed, or the chair and bounce up and down, or simply stay seated and perform your well rehearsed bumps and grinds. Again, he'll have easy access to your breasts and clitoris, and you to his scrotum. Never did a king sitting on his throne have so much fun!

183. *The upside-down position.* If you are both physically fit, this is a great one. You should lie face-down on the bed, legs hanging over the edge. He enters you from behind and helps you raise your legs and wrap them around his waist or shoulders. Or you can start on the floor; he lifts your ankles and holds them at his hip level while you walk around the floor on your hands! Besides the acrobatic fun of this elegant trick, it also makes for very deep penetration (some say the deepest) and lots of wild excitement. So what are you waiting for?

side by side

184. *The spoon.* Lie on your side in the semifetal position while your lover lies in the same position behind you, like two spoons curled up together. This position does not allow him to penetrate very deeply, but he *can* easily reach around to caress your clitoris and breasts. It's perfect for "sex and the single bed" and for sleepy early-morning lovemaking.

You can add some excitement to this position by grinding your bottom tantalizingly against his pelvis, raising your top leg over his to change the angle of entry, bending down at the waist to give him more direct and deeper access, massaging his behind with your free hand, or reaching through your legs to fondle the part of his penis that is not able to get inside you. And don't forget those sexy vaginal contractions you've learned to do; they'll drive him wild from any position.

185. *The scissors.* The basic scissors position is this: Lie on your back, have your man lie next to you on his side, and lift your leg over his. Both of you can move your legs around, entangling them in any position that gives you pleasure. One of my favorite leg positions involves maneuvering my body into a right angle from his and then raising my leg over his shoulder. This opens the vagina even wider and makes for lots of lovely genital contact for both parties.

The angle of entry created by the scissors position stimulates parts of his penis and scrotum that don't usually get that kind of attention; so it's a treat you should give him every once in a while. And since both of your hands are free, lightly scratch, tickle, knead, squeeze, or caress his manly chest, stomach, and legs. Though he won't be penetrating as deeply as he can in some other positions, he'll be too ecstatic to notice!

186. For a slightly different scissors, lie on your back with your legs raised while he places himself at a right angle under your legs. You can simply lower your legs when he enters, or he can put his top leg between yours. Again, both of you can and should get in all the fondling you can.

sitting face-to-face

187. Handy for sex in the tub, the kitchen, and other confined spaces, this is a position that allows for lots of visual and manual contact and playful or deep kissing. Simply sit face-to-face and wrap your legs around his waist. It works while sitting on the bed or floor, but he may have to support his weight by leaning back on his hands. For greater comfort, sit on a cushy chair or love seat. Then you'll both have your hands and lips free for adventure. You will have the most freedom of movement, so look him straight in the eye and undulate, rotate, and gyrate!

188. Remember that wonderfully salacious scene from *Last Tango in Paris*? They were sitting on the floor, face-to-face, having animalistic sex. It's not too difficult to make this work in your own "empty" apartment. You should both raise your knees, keeping feet flat on the floor, and lean back on straight arms. Once he's inserted in your highly excited vagina, you can rock forward and back, thrusting and retreating. Because your movements are somewhat contained, the best part of this position is the view you have of each other's genitals. Watching his glistening erection penetrate your pulsing vagina again and again is an incredibly sexy turn-on for any man — or woman.

189. For several years, I fantasized about being vigorously made love to by a man standing in front of me while I was seated on my dresser, legs hanging over the edge. But, in real life, I could never get all the body parts to come out in the right places, until one magic day, a man of just the right height finally fulfilled my fantasy. It was worth the wait!

But you don't have to wait to give yourself and your man one of the most delightful sex sessions you'll ever have. The secret is to find a surface to perch on that falls just below your man's crotch—the perfect height for proper insertion of penis A into slot B. This position has lots of advantages for your man—he doesn't have to support himself or you; he can thrust away wildly, un-encumbered by any body parts or weighty pressures; his hands are completely free and equally busy; he can shove his sword in up to the hilt; and he can easily feast his eyes on your jiggling tits and your luscious vagina devouring his eager erection. You will, of course, be enjoying the benefits of his deeply embedded penis and his pelvis slapping against you, his roaming hands, and your own view of the spectacular show.

And once you get the hang of it, you can take this show on the road—to the kitchen counter, dining room table, desk in your office, airplane bathroom, or any-where else you can think of. It's very convenient for sex on the move because very little disrobing is required, and this, in fact, adds a touch of urgency and secretly stolen pleasure to the occasion.

190. The windmill position is not a seated one, but since it must start out that way, I've included it here. Begin sitting face-to-face, your legs on top of his, penis

securely plugged in. Then both of you lie back flat on the bed, each person's upper body between the other's spreadeagled legs. You can either join hands or use them to play with each other's genitals, legs, and feet. Instead of thrusting, your pelvises should twist, knead, and undulate with varying rhythms and pressures. In this restful yet exciting situation, your man can stay hard for a long time—and keep you at the brink of orgasm indefinitely.

variations on the main theme

191. *The foot fetish.* During intercourse, whenever you're in a position to reach his feet easily, you might consider this little trick. Just as he's about to have his orgasm, grasp his toes and pull gently. It seems that a man's toe bone is connected to his genital bone, and this extra stimulation increases the intensity of his ejaculation.

192. *The taut tiger.* Keep your man's penile skin stretched tight the entire time you are having intercourse by holding it down with your fingers at the base. Imagine the heightened sensitivity you would experience if he stretched the skin around your exposed clitoris while thrusting against it with his pelvis, and you'll understand why this magic maneuver can send him skyward!

193. *Bondage (his).* Not for one-night stands, this should be done only with a man you know and trust and who trusts you. But once having established a certain degree of faith in each other, a little light bondage can be quite thrilling. Never leave anyone tied up for a long period of time or while you leave the room, though; you don't want to destroy the trusting relationship or the excitement.

After getting the okay from him, truss him up. Use silk scarves, his own necktie, soft ropes, your stockings, or anything else soft but strong enough to hold him. Fasten him, spreadeagled, to the bedposts, or simply tie his feet together and hands behind his head or back. Then tease him. Let him inhale your highly personal aroma. Caress and kiss him everywhere but his genitals. Brush your nipples and your pubic hair over his stomach, chest, and up to his mouth, but make him wait awhile before allowing him to lick you there. Take advantage of his helplessness by tonguing his underarms—a very sensuous undertaking that should leave him panting. Masturbate him. Suck his frantic penis. Play with him like a favorite toy. And then, at last, get on top of him, slip him inside, and thrust fast and passionately. Untie him right away as his post-orgasmic muscles will quickly get stiff. To put the icing on the cake, you might even massage the cramps out of his muscles and soothe him into a relaxed glow.

194. *Bondage (yours)*. Turnabout is fair play, and you'll give your man a powerful psychological thrill by letting him tie you up. His fantasies of controlling submissive little you will be excitingly brought to life. Again, this is to be done only with someone you trust completely. While he's teasing you, let your moans and groans tell him you can hardly bear the maddening pleasure he's inflicting. Undulate your pelvis provocatively (it's the only thing you can move anyway) and tell him you can't wait to have his gorgeous hard thing inside you. Beg him to put it in. When he does, you'll reap the benefit of his fever-pitch passion.

195. *Bondage variation (yours)*. Have him tie your hands together and feet together, then set you up on your elbows and knees. He then comes from behind to ravish you mercilessly while you love every minute of it!

196. *Oriental pearls*. Asian women are famous

for this fabulous trick. Sometime during foreplay, insert a string of beads (any beads will do, but pearls are very elegant) gently into his anus. It's a good idea to lubricate him with cream or oil first. Later, while he's busy thrusting, pull the pearls out one at a time and watch his passion mount. At the right moment, suddenly yank the rest of the string free and enjoy his explosive orgasm.

197. Slather each other with oil (baby oil, olive oil, petroleum jelly, or the like) and enjoy a smooth, slippery lovemaking session. Protect the sheets with towels or do it in the bathtub.

198. Don't relegate the vibrator to foreplay only. Give him a shattering orgasm by gliding the vibrator tip into his anus while you're happily humping away.

199. *Rock-a-bye baby.* Try doing it in a rocking chair. It's easier to use the armless variety, but any kind will do as long as you can both fit into it comfortably. He should sit in the chair so you can mount him and brace your feet on the rungs or on the floor. Just be careful your erotic enthusiasm doesn't tip the chair over!

200. Wetness and sex go hand in hand. So invite your man into the bathtub or shower, lather each other up, massage his slippery penis, and rub it up against your soapy pelvis and vaginal lips, and finally let him slide it in and out. *Do not* worry about getting your hair wet! Your skittishness will be a turn-off for him; and no matter how awful you think you look with wet hair, he'll think you're a very sexy mermaid!

201. Few things turn a man on more than a lusty woman showing him how much she's enjoying herself, how much his thrusting penis is turning her on. So let your passion show. Moan and groan with pleasure. Pant with excitement. Wriggle with abandon because you're so hot you just can't keep still. Nuzzle him appreciatively. Parry his thrusts eagerly. Wrap your legs around him and squeeze. Grab his bottom and push him into you with each thrust as if you can't get enough of him. Gently scratch and bite; he'll be proud to bear the scars of your passion. Vibrate. Scream. Grind. Toss and turn. Lick, kiss, and suck him as if you'd like to swallow him whole. Each move, each sound, each sensation will magnify his excitement and spur him on to even more fabulous lovemaking. And don't forget to . . .

202. *Tell* him how excited you feel. Earlier, I

touted the benefits of verbal foreplay, but now that the game is in full swing, you can really get down to talking "dirty." This is not the time for clinical descriptions of "vaginas" and "penises." This is the time to talk about "cocks," "pussies," and "fucking." These are perfectly wonderful words that we shouldn't feel ashamed to use. At the moment of passion, they are the most lovingly lascivious and appropriate words in the language. So get used to telling him how good it feels in every way you can think of.

- *"Honey, it's so good."*
- *"You're so hard."*
- *"You have the most gorgeous cock."*
- *"I love the feel of you in my pussy."*
- *"You make me so hot."*
- *"Fuck me, darling."*
- *"Fuck me harder (deeper, faster, etc.)"*
- *"Suck my tits."*
- *"I can't get enough of your dick."*
- *"My pussy is so wet for you."*
- *"Yes—more—deeper—harder!"*
- *"Give it to me."*
- *"Fill me up with your juice."*
- *"Please don't stop."*
- *"I love the way you fuck me."*
- *"I'm so hot for that big, beautiful prick."*
- *"Please put your gorgeous cock in my pussy."*
- *"Please let me fuck you."*

- *"Mmm, you're so wonderful, darling."*
- *"I love the feel of your beautiful long (thick, curved, strong, hard, bulging, smooth, ridgy, pulsing) dick thrusting in and out of me."*

Don't pay any false compliments. Find something about your guy that you can praise honestly, and do it, often and lovingly. Build up his sexual ego and he'll build up your sexual excitement. Sometimes the use of just one four-letter word is enough to stiffen his erection or make him come. So use some down-and-dirty words and you'll both get your sexual juices flowing.

203. *High-intensity orgasm.* You can give your man one of the most unforgettable experiences of his life—an orgasm that, like yours, involves shuddering spasms throughout his whole body. This takes time, patience, and concentration. Like you, the longer he is stimulated, the more intense his orgasm will be. So the secret to giving your man a high-intensity orgasm is to stretch out the period of buildup as long as possible by moving slowly and resting frequently. During regular intercourse, you won't have as much control over the pacing as you would if you were using only your hands or if he were tied up, but you can exert some control with your own slow thrusting or by saying something like, "Slower, darling. I want to make love to you for a long time."

With his penis inside you, it will also be more difficult for you to tell when he's almost at the point of no return. But as you get to know his sexual personality, you'll pick up clues. You may be able to feel him growing thicker and stiffer and his penile veins bulging out, or he may start panting or vibrating. At this critical point, make him stop thrusting and lie still for about ten seconds. You may even want to "unplug" him momentarily or use the squeeze technique (see page 25).

When he has calmed down, go back to what you were doing or try something else until he reaches the brink of orgasm again. Stop once more; you may want to extend this to a wine or talk break before you resume again. Don't make him stop more than three or four times or he may have trouble reaching an eventual orgasm. When you want him to finally have his high-intensity orgasm, increase the speed of your movements, twitch your sensuous vaginal muscles, and get serious about stroking and kissing him all over, especially on the ears, neck, underarms, and nipples. Although your man may resist this way of lovemaking at first, once he's tried it he'll beg you for more.

"Sexuality is not a leisure
or part-time activity. It is
a way of being."
—Alexander Lowen,
Love and Orgasm

6
it's all
in
your
head

I'm sure you know by now that there are many more than 203 ways to drive him wild in bed. You will invent endless variations on the themes I've presented here, especially when you and your man start improvising together. In the end, it's your own sensuous mind that's the best source of sexy new turn-ons and exotic man pleasers. So keep that cerebral sex muscle well exercised and vital!

Read lots of sex books, both how-to manuals and erotic tales. Imagine yourself doing all the wonderfully naughty things they suggest. Let yourself be carried away with your erotic dreams. Invent newer, more elaborate fantasies. Star in your own Technicolor porno flicks of the imagination. Pretend that you're Sophia Loren, or Marilyn Monroe, or Kathleen Turner, or whomever you think of as sex incarnate, and imagine what she would do to arouse her man.

Instead of walking down the street thinking of what to buy for dinner, check out all the attractive men you pass by. Notice the fit of their slacks. Picture how they would look naked. Try to imagine how they would move on top of you, how they would kiss you. Buy some magazines showing pictures of naked men. Ogle them privately. Go to a male stripper club and drink in all the sights. Let your imagination run wild!

Picture your own man — every rippling muscle, every manly hair, every soft and hard surface. Fantasize about what you're going to do to him tonight and how much he's going to love it. Imagine what he will do to you. Create the most sensuous scenario you can, including all the sights, sounds, smells, tastes, and textures. See yourself acting like the sexy, irresistible woman you know is inside of you. She's the woman who's going to drive her man wild in bed tonight and every night from now on.

Have a ball!

APPENDIX: GUIDELINES FOR

SAFER SEX

These guidelines were created by the Gay Men's Health Crisis (from their pamphlet *HIV & AIDS: The Basics* written by Stephen de Francesco, © Gay Men's Health Crisis, Inc.):

"Safer sex is just common sense. Since we know that the [HIV] virus is transmitted by body fluids entering another body, the sensible way to prevent infection is to block that entrance. *Latex condoms (rubbers) have been proven to be the most effective prevention against HIV infection.* Lambskin and other 'natural membrane' products are not as good as latex. They may allow HIV to pass through. The use of spermicidal (sperm-killing) lubricants, especially those with nonoxynol-9, may increase your protection. But they should always be used with a condom and never instead of a condom.

"Many condoms are prelubricated, some with spermicide, but you will probably want to use unlubricated condoms for oral sex with men. Condoms still provide the greatest protection, and relieve you of the worry about the risk involved. Both men and women should learn how to use condoms properly. Make them an integral part of sex and not an embarrassing, fumbling intermission.

"Here are the basic steps: When the penis is hard, roll the condom down all the way to the base, leaving some space at the head. Also, be sure to squeeze any air bubbles out. In vaginal or anal intercourse, *use plenty of water-based lubricant* . . . (baby oil, hand lotions, and petroleum-based products . . . can break down the latex within minutes). This will reduce the risk of breaking the rubber or injuring body tissue, which could leave an opening for infection.

"Condoms seldom break when used correctly, but it's still a good idea to [have your man] pull out before coming. The condom should be rolled off (not pulled) after coming and before losing the erection. Don't take the condom out of its sealed package until you're ready to put it on. And don't rip the package open with your teeth — you might rip the condom, too. Keep unopened condoms protected from heat, sunlight, moisture, and fluorescent light. Most companies put an expiration date on the box or on the individual wrappers. Others put the date of manufacture. When stored in a cool, dry place (not [a] wallet or glove compartment!) condoms are good for about two years from the date of manufacture. . . .

"In oral sex with women, dental dams may be used. (However, they have not been tested for protection against HIV.) A dental dam is a six-inch-square piece of thin latex that's available in dental and medical supply stores. *You can make a home-made dam by cutting a rolled condom to the center and opening it up.* In both cases, it should be rinsed first to remove any talc or other substance, and then dried. The dam should cover the entire vulva and should be held at both edges. Be careful not to turn the dam inside-out during oral sex, since this will totally defeat the purpose. Dental dams can also be used for oral-anal sex by both men and women. Remember: *Never reuse condoms or dental dams!!!*"

■   ■   ■

Remember, too, that even safer than latex barriers are activities like massage, hugging, body-to-body rubbing, mutual masturbation, dry kissing, fantasy, voyeurism, and exhibitionism. If you've read the rest of this book, you've learned some great techniques for making all those activities wonderfully erotic—and you've probably developed some of your own. Use and expand on these and never forget that great sex begins in your head (and heart). I've heard of couples who give each other orgasms merely by staring into each other's eyes!

Sex is not as carefree, and dare-free, as it used to be; but if you act wisely and responsibly, you and your man can still drive each other wild in bed.